AN EIGHT YEAR GOODBYE

A Memoir

Our Family's Journey on the Path of
Alzheimer's Disease

MARYANNE V. SCOTT

PAGE PUBLISHING, INC.
Conneaut Lake, PA

First originally published by Page Publishing 2020

ISBN 978-1-64701-985-3 (pbk)
ISBN 978-1-64701-987-7 (hc)
ISBN 978-1-64701-986-0 (digital)

Printed in the United States of America

This book is dedicated to all the caregivers caring for loved ones with Alzheimer's disease. You are the unsung heroes in this difficult battle.

CONTENTS

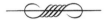

INTRODUCTION

The Roller Coaster

My father died on January 23, 2014, at 5:15 p.m. Well, his heart stopped beating, and he took his last breath at that time. So he physically died on that day at that moment. However, the father that I grew up with, the man who protected me and provided for me, who could fix anything, who could handle any situation, who was witty and sharp and strong and independent started to die eight years prior to that day in the fall of 2005. You see, my father had Alzheimer's disease, the cruel disease that robs a person of their mind, their thoughts, their precious memories. And the horrible disease that robs the victim's loved ones of the person that they knew.

It has been said that Alzheimer's disease is called "the long good-bye." I am here to tell you that it is a long goodbye that takes you on a roller-coaster ride of emotions each and every day and leaves you feeling exhausted and helpless. For my brother and I, it was an eight year goodbye filled with fear, sadness, confusion, anger, and loss.

There are over five million Americans living with Alzheimer's disease today and over sixteen million caregivers riding this emotional roller coaster. These caregivers are also saying goodbye to their loved ones—a long, painful goodbye. I've been in those shoes. I've been on that terrible ride. I said goodbye to my father a little bit each and every day from the fall of 2005 until he took his last breath in January 2014. It was a roller-coaster ride I couldn't wait to get off of. Here is my story.

CHAPTER 1

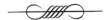

The Farm

My father, Samuel Valenti, was born on February 8, 1920, to two Italian immigrants named Felix and Maria Valenti. He had a large family with four older brothers, Charles, Frank, Anthony, and Joe, and an older sister, Theresa. His family lived in a small row home in Philadelphia, Pennsylvania, with his grandmother until he was twelve years old. At that time, his mother (the boss, as my father used to refer to her) got the brilliant idea to move to a farm in Mount Holly, New Jersey, to start a new life in farming. When my dad would tell me the story of this move, it would often remind me of the old TV show *Green Acres*, only in reverse. Where, on the show, the wife loved the city and the husband longed for the farming life, my grandfather was the city dweller, loving the excitement and activity, while my grandmother craved the solitude of the quiet New Jersey countryside. Since, as my father stated, my grandmother was the boss, the family found themselves on a 158-acre tomato farm in New Jersey, forcing everyone to take up the farming life. In my dad's words, "It was quite an adjustment."

This new life required Dad to do many things that he had never done before: plant and harvest crops, feed and care for the animals, and fix the farm equipment. He obviously had never had to tackle any of these chores in Center City, Philadelphia. Since he was still in school at the time of this move, the arrangement was for him to live with his grandmother in Philadelphia during the school year and go to the farm when school was over. However, the farming life interfered with the school year. So he would have to leave school a month early, in May, when the planting needed to be done and start a month late, in October, after the crops had all been harvested. This did not create the ideal atmosphere for academic success. He maintained this schedule until he reached tenth grade, which is when he dropped out of school to work full time on the farm.

Although Dad was used to the city life and had not initially chosen life on a farm, he grew to enjoy it. He and his brother, Joe, each had a horse and rode around the 158 acres when time permitted. His family owned cows, chickens, horses, and pigs. Dad went from never owning a pet while living in the city to owning an entire menagerie of pets on the farm. Dad's horse, Harry, was his favorite.

He spent many hours caring for Harry and exploring the farm with him. One day, they came upon a cow in the field that had passed away. Dad dismounted Harry and went to investigate. When he turned around to face Harry, he saw tears coming out of the horse's eyes. He began to view the farm animals as pets with feelings instead of just farm animals. But that didn't stop him and his family from eating some of their pets!

I used to ask him, when I was growing up, how he could eat the cows, pigs, and chickens that he fed, cared for, and talked to every day. This seemed so cruel to me. However, he stated that times were tough since it was during the Depression, and the family had to eat. So, many times, Dad would go into the barn, pet the animals that he cared for and then at night, they would eat one of them for dinner. It was definitely not what they would have done in the city.

One of the many advantages of farm life was eating the fresh crops that they planted. He and his brothers would go into the field, pick tomatoes off the vine, and sit down and eat them. They planted and harvested everything from tomatoes and corn to beans and melons. Even though it was the Depression, Dad's family ate very well.

The main reason that his mother wanted to move to a farm was so that they could make a prosperous living from it. They sold the tomatoes that they harvested to Campbell's Soup Company, which was in Camden, New Jersey. Although Dad's older brothers no longer lived at home, they would come back to assist with the harvesting. So between all the Valenti brothers, they were able to load up their Ford Model A pickup truck with the many bushels of tomatoes that they had picked by hand and haul the crop off to Camden. There were many trips made to and from the farm, but in the end, the fruits of their labor paid off, and they had enough money to get them through the year until the next crop was harvested.

On May 6, 1937, late in the day, Dad was working in the fields, tilling the earth to get it ready for planting. Suddenly, he saw a very large shadow crossing overhead. The shadow seemed to go on forever. When he looked up, he realized that it was the Hindenburg making its transatlantic flight from Frankfurt, Germany, to Lakehurst, New Jersey, twenty-five miles away from Dad's farm. Dad watched in awe as the airship sailed overhead, looking like he could reach up and touch it. He watched it sail until he could no longer see the amazing sight and then went back to tilling the earth. A short time later, his mother ran out into the field to tell him that she had just heard that the Hindenburg had blown up. In shock and disbelief, his family huddled by the radio to learn the details of this horrific event.

Many of Dad's extended family came to spend time with them on the farm. Both of his parents had brothers and sisters, so there were many cousins who came to enjoy the farm life. Two of their frequent visitors were Dad's cousin, Mildred Italiano, and her daughter, Anna. Dad enjoyed when little Anna came over, and he loved showing her all the farm animals. Anna always loved Dad and remembered him later in life when she became the Academy Award-winning actress, Anne Bancroft. She helped him earn brownie points with his future wife many years later when she invited them backstage after her performance in *The Miracle Worker* on Broadway!

Dad slowly transformed from a city dweller to a farmer over the years that he worked on the farm. There were many aspects of farming life that he had to learn and one area, in particular, that he became very adept at. That was repairing the farm equipment. I remember stories from my aunts and uncles about how mechanically inclined Dad was. No matter what the machine was—tractor, tiller, feed grinder—he could take it apart and put it back together and have it working as good as new.

His father, seeing Dad's potential and talent, decided that Dad needed to further his education. His dream was to see his son go to school for engineering. As I stated, the year was around 1937, which was during the Great Depression. While Dad's family was not destitute like so many families were at that time, they were by no means prosperous enough to afford higher education. But that did not stop Felix from repeatedly proclaiming, "I don't know how I'm going to do it, but I'm going to send you to school. I'm not going to see that talent go to waste."

On the evening of December 29, 1938, Maria and Felix had an argument. Felix went for a long walk as he often did when he needed to think and cool down. He was walking along Route 206, which is where they lived, maybe thinking about the argument, maybe wondering how he was going to pay for Dad's education, when he was struck by an eighteen-wheel tractor trailer. He was killed instantly.

I remember Dad telling me the story about someone knocking on their door with the news and how for the next four days, his dad's body was laid out in a casket in their living room for family and friends to come and view. I also remember him saying that he realized that, without his dad there, all the farming responsibilities were now going to fall on he and his brother Joe. I'm sure, at this point, he also realized that any thoughts and dreams of higher education died along with his father. He was now going to have to stay on the family farm.

CHAPTER 2

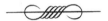

The War

Dad continued to work on the farm until March of 1944. At that time, he received his draft notice from the United States Army. He was now entering World War II at twenty-four years old and heading to Europe.

He began basic training at Fort Knox in Kentucky. I remember him telling me about how arduous the training was, from getting up at the crack of dawn to run twenty-five miles with heavy backpacks on, to having to do push-ups until he felt like he was going to throw up. When I would ask him how he did it, he would reply that "you did what you had to do." He was in terrific shape already from all the manual labor that he had to do on the farm. But he knew he had to get in even better condition if he was going to go defend his country, which he felt honored to do. He left for Germany in May of 1944 and joined Company L of the 320th Infantry Division of the United States Army.

Growing up, I could tell that Dad never liked to talk about the war. Whenever I would ask him questions, he would quickly change the subject. However, on the rare occasions that he did open up, the stories were horrendous. There was the time that he and a few of his fellow soldiers took cover from the raining mortar shells one pitch-black night in an abandoned building. Upon waking up the next morning, they realized that they were surrounded by dead bodies. Or the time that he and his best friend from their days in basic training together were running through a field, and his friend was blown up right next to him. Dad was knocked out, and when he came to, he found his rifle bent in half from the explosion of the bomb and pieces of his friend's body scattered on the ground.

On another occasion, he told the story of marching across a freshly plowed field at night. The soldiers were having difficulty walking because of the soft dirt, but they kept moving forward as best they could. As they were gaining ground, the soldiers in the lead set off a trip wire, and flares were sent up that lit up the sky as if it were daylight. Their sergeant started yelling for everyone to run, and Dad began running in a zigzag pattern as bullets were hitting the ground near his feet. When he got to the other side of the field, he dove into a foxhole to take cover. As he lifted his head to see what was happening, he came face-to-face with a German soldier lying on the ground, holding a rifle pointed at him. Dad's life passed before his eyes as he realized this was the end for him. When the soldier didn't fire, Dad crept forward and saw that the soldier was dead with the top of his head having been blown off. This was one of the many times that he came eye to eye with death.

However, the most awful of Dad's war stories was the time that, again, to escape enemy fire, he dove into a foxhole, and the shrapnel from an exploding hand grenade hit him in the back and was embedded into him. He was taken to an emergency field hospital, and ten of the twenty-eight pieces of shrapnel were removed. The other eighteen pieces remained there for the rest of his life. The doctors told him they could not remove any more of the pieces because they were too close to his lung, and it was too dangerous. (This made for some interesting conversation whenever we went through metal detectors at airports when I was growing up!)

When Dad was brought to the emergency field hospital, he was separated from his division. Due to this, he was declared "missing in action." I remember as a little girl seeing the letter that was sent to my grandmother from the United States government. The letter said, "We regret to inform you that your son, Private First-Class Samuel Valenti, is Missing in Action. We have no further information at this time." I couldn't imagine how horrible it would be for a mother to receive a letter like that. Dad remained at the field hospital until he had sufficiently recovered from his wounds and then was reunited with his division.

Dad fought in the war from March of 1944 until he was honorably discharged on November 19, 1945. He received a Purple Heart Medal, a Bronze Star Medal, and a Good Conduct Medal for his services during the war. He also received many commendation letters for the successful battles that his division fought from majors and generals. He always downplayed his medals and achievements whenever anyone brought them up because he was a very humble man. However, throughout the rest of his life, he was always proud to tell everyone that he served his country in World War II. And he was extremely patriotic, displaying the American flag at his homes and getting visibly emotional whenever he stood with his hand on his heart during the "Star-Spangled Banner." He was truly proud to be an American.

CHAPTER 3

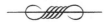

Coming Home

After Dad was honorably discharged from the United States Army in November 1945, he arrived home a few weeks later to an empty house. From stories that I had heard about my grandmother, she was not a very warm and fuzzy kind of mother. I would have had banners, flags, and a feast waiting for my returning soldier son. However, upon his return, everyone was out and about doing their own thing. I could tell from the way Dad told the story that it was a very disappointing homecoming.

When my brother and I were growing up, my mother, who was the definition of warm and fuzzy, turned every occasion into a celebration. Our birthdays were observed with our favorite meals, a homemade cake, streamers, and presents. Every holiday was a feast. My father would say to my mother, "Why do you make such a big deal about it? It's just another day." As I got older, I asked him how his birthday and holidays were celebrated, and he said that they weren't. His mother did none of the elaborate things that my mother did. She treated it as "just another day." So I guess that's how she treated her son's return from the war…as just another day.

After the war, Dad took advantage of the GI Bill and went to school for welding. He was finally able to get the education that he was deprived of when his father died years ago. He graduated from welding school and immediately started working at multiple jobs "fixing things," which he was so talented at doing.

One of the first purchases that Dad made with the money he was now earning was a new Harley-Davidson motorcycle. I used to hear the stories from my aunts and uncles about my father riding around town on his Harley, and I just couldn't picture it. I think most people can not picture their parent as a young, vibrant, carefree, biker. I only saw him as a responsible, conscientious, hardworking man. But as I was growing up, he always used to say whenever he saw a motorcycle go by, "I used to have a bike, a Harley. I loved to ride." And I'd chuckle under my breath at the image of my dad with his hair blowing in the wind as he tore around on his hog.

Growing up, I had known that Dad lived at home on the farm until he married my mom when he was forty years old! I thought that it was a little strange that he lived home with his mother all that time. Then I realized that he stayed there to continue to help her with the farm. His older siblings had moved out, and my grandmother was there alone. So not only did he hold down a full-time welding job (working whatever overtime hours he could to earn more money) but he also worked on the farm. This schedule certainly did not leave much time for anything else, especially dating.

CHAPTER 4

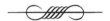

The Romantic

In February 1959, Dad was thirty-nine years old and still not married or involved in a serious relationship. My aunts used to say that they could not understand why a woman had not latched onto him yet because he was so handsome and such a wonderful man. I wonder if Dad wasn't interested because of the responsibility that he felt to my grandmother and the farm.

Occasionally on Saturday nights, Dad would go to a dance hall in Philadelphia called Wagner's. At that time, dance halls were where young people went to socialize. There were many of them in Philadelphia, but Dad had not been to Wagner's in a while, so he decided to venture there one Saturday night in February of 1959. He was standing near a wall when a woman came up and stood behind him. He turned around and asked her to dance. That woman was my mother.

My mother, Mary Dellose, was at Wagner's that particular weekend against her will. Apparently, she and her unmarried friends would go there every week in the hopes of meeting an eligible bachelor. This particular evening, she was reluctant to go. She had her fill of going there to try to meet a nice guy. However, her friends talked her into going, and she went, halfheartedly. She noticed a man who she had met previously and did not particularly care for, so in an attempt to avoid him, she hid behind another man standing by the wall. A rather handsome man at that! After a few minutes, this gentleman turned around and asked her to dance. That man was my father.

Apparently, they talked all night, and my father must have made a profound impression on my mother because when she left, she told her friends, "I'm going to marry that guy." My mother was thirty-seven at the time and had also never been married. According to my grandfather, it was because she was "too goddamned picky." She had dated many different men over the years but had found something wrong with all of them. They were too tall, too short, too fat, too thin, they smoked, they drank, etc. On that night in February 1959, she had found the perfect man.

Mom and Dad dated all throughout that spring, summer, and into the fall. When Mom would tell me stories of their courtship, I was always struck by how "in love" she sounded when she talked about it. However, to me, who was full of romantic notions of what a love affair should be, he did not sound like a very romantic partner.

Dad never brought her flowers, wrote her love notes, or planned romantic rendezvous. He just showed up at her parents' house (she also still lived at home) in Pennsylvania every Saturday night to take her out to dinner or just hang out. He never called her during the week; he just arrived at her house. It did not matter to Mom though. She thought he was the perfect man. He didn't drink in excess, smoke, or gamble. Those were her parameters. And my grandparents loved him. He would show up many times on a Saturday night and go down to the basement with my grandfather to sample some of his homemade wine. My father and grandfather would sit in the basement, drinking the wine and eating pepperoni and cheese while Mom would be upstairs waiting for him. After these encounters, my grandfather would tell my mom to keep her mouth shut and not do anything to mess up this relationship because she had such a good guy. He was a typical old-fashioned Italian father.

One exciting date Dad did plan for them was the time Dad took her to New York City to see *The Miracle Worker* on Broadway. Dad's cousin, Anne Bancroft, was performing in the award-winning play, and Dad had gotten tickets. After the play was over, Dad suggested that they go backstage to see Anne. When they tried to go to her dressing room, they were stopped by the guard. When he asked just what they thought they were doing, Dad replied, "I'm Anne's cousin, and we wanted to stop and congratulate her on her performance."

"Yeah, yeah, that's what they all say," said the guard.

"No, really," Dad replied. "Go tell Anne that her cousin Sam from Mount Holly is here. I'm sure she'll want to see me."

The gentleman reluctantly did as my dad asked. Moments later, Anne came running out, threw her arms around Dad, and hugged and kissed Mom. Then she invited them into her dressing room for a visit. Mom was starstruck and very impressed. Dad had won some brownie points that evening.

Despite her father's advice to keep her mouth shut, Mom just couldn't. Christmas of 1959 came and went, and Mom had hoped that they would get engaged. They had been dating for ten months, and they were in love. They were older and did not have time to waste if they were going to have a family. So she discussed this with him in January. She laid it on the line and basically told him to "shit or get off the pot."

Unfortunately, it did not go over well. She did not hear from Dad for the next three weeks. She waited for him to call, but he never did. Saturday nights came and went, and he never showed up. This was before Facebook and social media, so she had no idea what he was doing. She had no way to stalk him. She also did not have his phone number, so she wasn't able to call him. She was devastated. While she wanted to push him along to make a decision about their future, she had not wanted to push him away entirely. Her "perfect" man was gone. And her father was furious that she had not kept her mouth shut!

One Saturday night at the beginning of February, Dad showed up at Mom's house unexpectedly. He sat her down and gave her what I assume he felt was a romantic marriage proposal. He said, "Well, I have some vacation time coming up in August, so why don't we get married then?" Just the kind of proposal that every girl dreams of! But for Mom, it was the happiest day of her life.

They went shopping for an engagement ring the following week. He told her to pick out whatever ring she wanted. After that lame proposal, most women would have picked out the largest diamond in the jewelry store. But Mom was never flashy or materialistic, so she picked out a modest diamond and was so proud to show it off to everyone. The plans were under way for their August 6 wedding when Dad had vacation time coming up.

CHAPTER 5

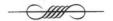

Family Life

Mom and Dad got married on August 6, 1960; she was thirty-eight, and he was forty. Mom's goal was to get pregnant right away. So I have a feeling that they were rather busy from then until January when they got pregnant with me. I was born in October 1961, and Mom said it was one of the happiest days of her life. But I think she had really wanted to give Dad a son. I had been told a story of my father and another new dad in the maternity ward waiting room, discussing the fact that they both had girls, and Dad's comment was, "Well, what are we going to do…we can't send them back?" My father had a way with words! Even though he had made this comment, expressing his obvious disappointment at not having had a son, over our many years together, it became obvious that I was the light of my father's life and, in his words, his "baby doll."

Soon afterward, Mom set out to get pregnant again even though her doctor warned her not to have any more children. Not only was Mom nearing forty, but she also had a heart condition. When she was two years old, she had rheumatic fever, which left her heart damaged. Her doctor felt that her advanced age and damaged heart would be problematic for her. He felt that the trauma of childbirth on her heart would be dangerous. However she did not listen. She wanted to give Dad a son.

My brother was born on May 31, 1963, two months premature. He died on June 1, 1963, fourteen hours after his birth. Mom could not go to his funeral because she was still in the hospital, recovering. My aunts and uncles were there with Dad as he carried my brother's little white casket. According to my uncle, my father's brother, it was the first time he had seen my dad cry. He was devastated.

Mom, once again, set out to get pregnant. This time, her doctor was adamant about her not getting pregnant. So she left his practice and found a doctor who would support her and help her accomplish her dream.

Mom got pregnant again and gave birth to my brother Sam in March 1965. She was almost forty-three, and Dad was forty-five. Dad was on top of the world—he finally had his son. I assume he didn't want to send *him* back!

Life in our household was the typical old-fashioned "Leave it to Beaver" household. Mom cooked, cleaned, ironed, and raised the kids. However, she did not wear a dress and pearls while doing all this like June Cleaver. Dad worked and earned the money to support the family financially.

I have wonderful memories of growing up in our family. We took many trips together to the Jersey shore, amusement parks, museums, parks, and lakes. Many of these trips were only day trips because Dad usually only had one day off from work. But we made the most of it and had fun no matter what we were doing.

Dad was very involved in our lives growing up. He always went to our back-to-school nights, taking a considerable interest in our education. He also was the teacher in our house, teaching us how to ride our bikes, how to cut the grass with the riding lawn mower, how to drive, and how to parallel park. But he was a "no holds barred" kind of guy when it came to that. There was no such thing as training wheels when he taught us how to ride our bikes. You got on the bike, and he held you while he gave you a push, and then once you started pedaling, he let you go. If you fell down, you were supposed to get right back up and try again. That method worked well for me. However, it did not work so well for Sam.

He decided to teach Sam how to ride his bike on the grass so that if he fell, he would not get hurt. He held onto him and the bike while Sam pedaled and, running alongside, let go when he got started. However, when he let him go, Sam steered directly into a tree. That was the end of the lesson for a while.

Dad used the same strategy when he taught us how to drive. He took us to abandoned parking lots to practice when we were fifteen, even before we had our permits. Once we got our permits at sixteen, we did not start out on lonely, deserted back roads. Dad took us out on the highway and told us to keep up with the flow of traffic! Dad went by the "sink or swim" philosophy of teaching his children.

One skill that Dad taught us that, to this day, I silently thank him for each time I do it, is how to parallel park. He drilled in to us the importance of learning the correct way to parallel park, which was to back in to the spot, not pull in. He would set up cones in a parking lot and make us practice over and over until we got it right. Due to his diligent teaching, I was able to parallel park my enormous Ford Expedition expertly in later years.

Dad was also very accommodating to most things that we wanted as we were growing up. I remember wanting a swing set when I was young and asking Dad to put one up for us. I assumed that he would go to our local toy store, Kiddie City, purchase a swing set, and put it together. That was not Dad's style. We had two huge oak trees in our yard that were about fifteen feet apart. Dad wedged a round, steel beam between the immense branches of the two trees and then welded four swings onto the beam. We had the unrivaled, best swing set in the entire neighborhood that was the envy of all the neighborhood kids.

I say that Dad was accommodating to most things because there was one item in particular that I continually asked for that Dad would not agree to. And he found an ingenious way to silence me for good. We had a very large backyard at our childhood home. A yard that would have been perfect for an in-ground swimming pool. Due to the fact that my mother did not drive, we spent our summers playing in our yard every day—every hot day. So I started my campaign of asking for a pool. Mom gave me all the usual reasons that we could not have one; they are too much work (I said I would help with the work), a neighborhood child could fall in (I said we could get a fence), and we would not use it after the novelty wore off (I swore

I would use it every day of the summer). Then one day, Dad said, "Maryanne, we can't put a pool in because our yard has a very steep slope. All the water would flow out." I obviously was not very bright at this point in my life because I begrudgingly accepted this fact and never asked about the pool again.

Another memory I have of our household as I was growing up was that it was a typical Italian household. We had homemade pasta with meatballs and sausage a few times a week. Mom and Dad canned tomatoes every August, which Mom used to make home-made spaghetti sauce, or gravy as we Italians call it. And whenever my parents wanted to talk about something that they did not want Sam and I to know about, they started speaking in Italian so that we could not understand what they were saying. It was very annoying.

Mom and Dad had a very strong work ethic. They believed that you work hard and save your money. While Mom was not employed outside the home, she did her part in scrimping and saving so that they were able to buy whatever it was that Sam or I needed. And Dad worked extremely hard at his job, picking up double shifts whenever the opportunity arose.

Dad's job was very grueling. He was a welder/steamfitter. I remember as a child seeing him come home from work soaking wet from sweat and filthy dirty after working outside in ninety-five degree weather, wearing an asbestos suit and steel mask to protect him from the flames from the welding torch. He would stagger in the door and immediately head into the shower where he would stay for about thirty minutes. Then he would sit down to dinner, talk to us about our day, and fall asleep in his recliner.

Some of the many places that he worked included naval ship yards, nuclear power plants, bridges, and metal fabrications facilities. Many of his welding jobs required Dad to climb to extremely high heights, which made Mom a nervous wreck. He worked outside in the freezing cold, extreme heat, rain, sleet, and wind. And he was not exactly a young man at this time. But he never complained and never missed a day of work. His work ethic was amazing.

While Dad made a decent living, he was not earning what he could have been had he been in a union. So he decided to take a test to get into the Steamfitters Union. He came home one day with a book that looked very intimidating. It was a very large technical book, and apparently, Dad needed to read it, study, and take an exam. Our lives were about to become difficult.

Every night, Dad would come home, take his thirty-minute shower, eat dinner, and lock himself in his bedroom to study. Sam and I were not permitted to make a sound. Mom would tell us repeatedly that Dad needed quiet and that this test was very important. So we would watch TV practically on mute and whisper to each other. The same thing went on all weekend as Dad would be locked in his bedroom studying. This went on for months. Finally, the big day came. We were now able to watch TV with the volume up. And Dad was taking the test.

I remember waiting anxiously for weeks to hear whether Dad had passed or not. Mom and Dad were nervous, and Dad looked exhausted. He had worked extremely hard for so many months. I remember praying that he passed, even if I did not quite understand the importance of this test.

Dad came home a few weeks later, beaming. He had passed the test and was now a member of the Steamfitters Union! We all hugged and congratulated him and told him how proud we were of him. Life became financially much better for us after that, as Dad was now making triple the money that he had made before joining the union. His jobs were still grueling and backbreaking for him, but he did not seem to mind them as much knowing that he was now making a very prosperous living doing it. We still had a typical "Leave it to Beaver" household, but we were now much more financially secure thanks to Dad passing that exam.

Due to our better financial status, we now were able to enjoy the finer things in life. Mom and Dad's first purchase was a color television set. We had previously had a black-and-white TV, so this was quite a step up for our family. I still remember going to shop for it and getting our large Zenith console color television. We all sat in awe, watching the beautiful colors on the screen. Shortly after getting the new television, we had central air-conditioning installed in our house. Previously, we had not had that luxury, and to keep cool in the unbearable heat of the summers, we would live in our basement. So having central air-conditioning was a luxury like no other. Along with this, my parents purchased a new car that also had air-conditioning. No more sticking to the hot leather seats and praying for a windy day so that we could get a breeze while driving. I remember thinking that we were rich. The quality of our life had significantly improved since Dad had passed that test. It was worth the many quiet nights that Sam and I had to endure.

While our household was typical in many ways, there was one area of our life that was not very commonplace and that I did not realize until much later in my life. This was Dad's abilities as a handyman. He could fix anything, just like when he was on the farm. There was not an appliance, bicycle, car, gadget, etc. that he could not take apart, replace the broken part, and then put back together.

Dad would come home from work, and Mom would say, "Sam, the washing machine is making a funny noise." The next thing we knew, he would be on the floor with pieces of the washer spread out all around him. Then he would be out the door to go buy the piece that he needed. And when he came back, miraculously, all the parts would be put back where they belonged, and the washer was working perfectly without the "funny noise."

This happened with just about anything in our house that was broken. It never occurred to me that other dads were not able to "fix" things as easily until one of my best friends told me that whenever anything was broken in their house, they had to call someone in to repair it. I took it for granted that Dad was so talented and mechanically inclined. We had our own personal handyman!

I remember coming home one day and describing to Dad a problem that I was having with my car. I said, "Dad, my car is making a rattling sound, doesn't accelerate when I step on the gas, and it smells like rotten eggs."

He immediately said, "Oh, that sounds like your catalytic converter."

Huh? What the heck was that? I thought. All I knew about cars was that you turned the key, stepped on the gas, and it moved. I had no idea what a catalytic converter was. Obviously, Dad did. He immediately went outside to take a look.

When I went outside a half hour later, parts were strewn all over the driveway. Dad was under the car, and strange noises were coming from that direction. A little while later, he hopped in his car to go off to Bob's Auto Parts Store. When he returned, he disappeared under my car again. Some more strange noises followed, and soon parts were being put back together.

He instructed me to start up the car and drive it around the block. Alas, no more rattling noise or rotten egg odor. And when I stepped on the accelerator, the car moved. Our handyman did it again. He was amazing.

Another characteristic I remember about Dad when I was growing up was how laid back and even-keeled he was. Not many situations rattled him. He was a kind and gentle man who rarely raised his voice and never raised his hand to Sam and I—well, almost never.

My brother and I grew up in a time when disciplining children with a slap, or in our case, a fly swatter was common place. Mom was the disciplinarian in our house. She was the yeller, the giver of dirty looks, and the wielder of the dreaded green fly swatter. Whenever we did anything wrong, she would open the door to the staircase that led down to the basement, take the fly swatter off the hook that it hung on, and proceed to smack us on the rear end with it. Granted, it wasn't as painful as a belt, which some of my friends were disciplined with, but it still stung.

When we were younger, Sam and I would just stand there and accept our punishment. However, as we got older, we became wiser. We realized that, because of Mom's heart condition, she was unable to run or climb stairs quickly. So we began to use this to our advantage. We would run up the stairs to the second floor, and Mom was not able to catch us. We would stay upstairs in our bedrooms until she calmed down and forgot what our offense was and then quietly sneak back downstairs when we felt it was safe. This strategy worked every time, and we were saved from the evil fly swatter on numerous occasions. Unfortunately, for us, that strategy did not work with Dad.

One day, when I was about fourteen and Sam was eleven, Dad was waiting for a very important work-related phone call. He told us ahead of time that he needed us to be quiet while he was on the call. At that time, there was no such thing as a portable phone. Our phone was stationary on a stand near the living room—right next to where Sam and I were watching television and arguing loudly about what to watch.

The phone rang, and Dad answered it with a look at us that said, "Be quiet." We were…for about the first two minutes of his phone call. Then we began arguing again. Mom was waving her arms at us and shooting us with those dirty looks that usually worked. Dad's face was becoming angrier as he was trying to write down information from the call that he obviously could not hear over the sounds of our bickering. I tried to quiet down, but Sam was being difficult, and I wanted my way. I was the oldest and always wanted my way. We continued to get increasingly louder.

Finally, Dad's phone call was over. We saw him hang up and turn around to look at us with a murderous look that we had never seen on Dad's face before. We knew we were in deep trouble. So we took off for the stairs. Fortunately for Dad, but unfortunately for us at that moment, Dad did not have a heart condition. So our fail-safe plan did not work with him.

I was ahead of Sam on the stairs. I turned halfway up the staircase to see him get a hard smack on the rear end. I reached the top of the stairs and thought that I was home free. Mom would never have made it up this far. I soon found out that I was sadly mistaken. As I got to the top step and rounded the corner of the long hallway, Dad reached out and slapped me on the back. The momentum of both of us running and the smack caused me to go flying down the hallway. I wasn't hurt, but I was astonished. First, because Dad had never hit us up until this point in my life. And secondly, that for such an old guy (he was fifty-five at the time, which was ancient to me), he could really move fast.

Dad went downstairs without a word to either of us. Sam and I sat upstairs trying to figure out where our system had failed. Mom came up to see us a little while later and told us that Dad felt terrible that he had hit us. That made us feel even worse.

We ended up apologizing to Dad, which we had never done after Mom disciplined us. We could tell that he felt horrible for what he had done even though Sam and I were definitely in the wrong. That was the first and last time that Dad had ever laid a hand on us. For the rest of his life, I would always just remember him as a gentle, kind, loving man.

CHAPTER 6

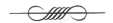

Ahead of His Time

I grew up in a very conflicted household. I don't mean that in the way you might think. My parents got along wonderfully, we all loved and supported each other, and aside from the typical family squabbles and disagreements, everything was very harmonious. However, my parents had conflicting views on what they wanted for me.

My mother graduated from high school in 1939 and found employment right out of school. She worked as a secretary for a bank and was content with her job. At that time, not many people attended college, and especially not women. While my mother was very intelligent and would most likely have done extremely well in college, the thought would never have crossed her mind to spend the kind of money that a college education would have cost. She and her family had lived and struggled through the Great Depression, so I'm sure, as soon as she was able, she wanted to get a job and earn money to help her family financially. Also, her goals in life were to get a job, find a nice man, get married, and raise a family. Unfortunately for her, this did not happen until 1960 when she met my dad.

Once she and Dad got married, she set out to achieve her goals of having children and being a stay-at-home mom. She made her husband, children, and home her primary focus. She was content with her role in life and excelled at this job. As a result, she felt that I should pursue the same path in life.

My father, on the other hand, was ahead of his time. He felt that education, whether for a man or a woman, was extremely important. I surmise that he felt this way due to the fact that he was not able to further his own education because of his father's premature death and his need to work on the family farm. He preached the importance of higher education to me my whole life, and he was willing to pay any amount for me to get it.

When I was in high school, I was not sure if I wanted to attend college. Since I was so unsure, Mom suggested that I attend a secretarial school and see if I had any interest in that as a career. Dad, on the other hand, suggested that I start college and give it a try. Of course, there was no talk of taking out student loans, as Mom and Dad insisted that they were going to pay for my education. When I said that I did not want to start college and waste their money if I did not continue, Dad stated, "Education is never a waste of money. Whether you finish or not, you are still obtaining knowledge." I decided to try community college for two years to see if I liked it.

I did very well in college and decided to continue on and complete my bachelor's degree. At one point, I became interested in law. I had taken a few law courses and loved them. I also argued with everyone about everything, so I felt that that characteristic could serve me well as a lawyer. I decided to discuss this new career idea with my parents one day and received very opposing opinions.

"How can you be a lawyer and stay home with your children some day?" Mom asked. "What kind of mother will you be with a career like that?"

Dad said, "That's great. Finish college and then go to law school. Let me know how much it is. I'll pay for all of it. Get as much education as you can."

This drew dirty looks and glares from Mom.

It was not until many years later that I realized how ahead of his time Dad was. For a man who grew up and struggled during the Great Depression, there was never any question or reservations about spending thousands of dollars on my education. And for a man growing up in a time when not many women went to college or had careers, he was thoroughly supportive of education, whether you were a man or a woman.

I did end up graduating from college with a bachelor's degree in business administration from Temple University, but I did not go on to law school. That interest faded although I do still argue about everything! Of course, Dad paid for my entire college education. As my friends were all talking about how they were going to pay off their student loans, I did not have a penny to repay. Dad was extremely proud of me for being the first person in his large family to ever graduate from college.

I do not know if I ever really appreciated his encouragement at the time or thanked him for believing in me, pushing me, and supporting me. He was always my biggest cheerleader, and I know he was very proud of my accomplishments. I'm thankful to my father to this day for being such an advocate for education and encouraging me every step of the way.

CHAPTER 7

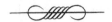

My Husband

I met my husband, Jim, when I was a junior in high school. They say you fall for guys that are similar to your father. That was true in my case. Jim was a kind, caring, respectful gentleman. Because that was the kind of man that I had grown up with, that is what attracted me to him. That and the fact that he was very handsome! Now he just had to pass my father's test.

While my father was always hospitable whenever I brought anyone new to our house, there was one feature about him that caused me to become nervous whenever I did bring someone over for the first time. Dad was very old-fashioned and believed wholeheartedly in respect. He felt that when someone came into his house, they should look him in the eye and address him. Most of my friends did this, and he always made them feel comfortable because they passed his requirements. He especially loved my childhood friend, Debbie, who always came in and said, "Hi, Mr. Valenti. How are you?" Many times, she would sit and have a long conversation with him, which he thoroughly enjoyed. Debbie spent a significant amount of time at our house when we were growing up, and both of my parents loved her. Since Debbie's respectfulness was the type of encounter Dad grew used to, when I brought a friend home that did not exhibit this same type of behavior, it did not go over very well with him.

One evening, one of my friends from college came to pick me up before we went out for the night. When she came in, I introduced her to my parents, and she barely said hello. My mother was friendly and made her feel welcome. My father, on the other hand, did not speak to her. I was mortified. We left shortly afterward, and I made excuses for my dad's behavior—he wasn't feeling well, he was tired, etc. It didn't seem to faze her, but I was furious with Dad.

When I spoke to him about it the next day, he was adamant about his rules. "When someone comes into my house, they need to address me and show respect," he proclaimed. Thereafter, whenever this particular friend came to my house, Dad barely spoke to her. It was very embarrassing, but I came to accept that it was Dad's house, and those were his rules. I thought about this when I brought Jim over to meet my parents for the first time. And I was nervous.

I should have prepped Jim before he walked in, but I did not think I needed to. I was right. He walked in and went right up to my father, looked him in the eye, shook his hand, and told him how good it was to meet him. Then he hugged my mother and said the same to her. My parents were hooked.

Jim proceeded to make conversation with my parents and was extremely respectful. He told my parents where we were going for the evening and when he would have me home. As we were leaving, he again shook my dad's hand and hugged my mother. They were in love.

Jim and I dated for eight years. My parents fell deeper in love with him each year. He was always invited for our Sunday midday meal of spaghetti and meatballs. If he was late getting out of church, we either had to wait for him to get there, or Mom would put a big plate aside for him. Jim had an old Volkswagen beetle while we were dating that was in desperate need of repair. When we first started seeing each other, the car did not have a passenger seat, and I had to sit on the floor when we went out. My parents were actually fine with this arrangement because I was with Jim. He could do no wrong in their eyes.

Many times, while we were dating, Jim and I did not go out anywhere. He would come over, and we would sit with my parents and Sam, watch TV, and order a pizza. My mother always rolled out the red carpet whenever he came over. And, of course, because he was so respectful, Dad just loved him. He easily became part of the family.

When Jim decided to propose to me, he, of course, did the right thing and went to ask my father's permission. This was the icing on the cake in terms of respect for my father. Dad gave his blessing, and Mom cried. They were ecstatic that Jim would now officially be part of our family. They could not have imagined a more perfect son-in-law.

We began the wedding preparations, and my father spared no expense. He planned to pay for the entire wedding and wanted me to have anything that I wanted. I had grown up with a mother that was very frugal and conscious of spending money, so I was going to try to keep the expenses down. That is, until I found my dream wedding gown.

The very first gown I tried on was exactly what I wanted, but the price was exorbitant. While Mom cried when she saw me in it and loved the dress, there was no way she could justify paying that kind of price for something that I was going to wear for eight hours. We proceeded to go to about ten other stores over the course of the next month, but nothing came close to that dress. I attempted to like one of the countless number of gowns I tried on, but nothing compared.

Being a typical man, Dad did not take part in any of the wedding minutiae. He just wrote the checks whenever we needed him to. But one day, he did ask if I had found a wedding gown yet. I told him about my endless search for something that would compare to my dream dress. His response was, "Why are you looking for something else if you have already found something that you love?" When I told him the price, he did not bat an eye. He simply said, "Get the gown. I want you to have whatever you want for your big day." I threw my arms around him and cried tears of happiness while my mother rolled her eyes. Then we headed out to get the dress of my dreams.

I did feel guilty about spending that kind of money, but I got over the guilt when I tried it on again. I tried to keep the expenses down in all the other aspects of the wedding. But Dad never complained and just kept writing the checks.

We had a beautiful wedding despite the torrential downpour that day. I remember Dad running to the hardware store that morning to get paint tarps to hold over me and all the bridesmaids so that we could get out to the cars without getting drenched. I remember feeling like a princess in my beautiful wedding gown. I also remember the proud look on Dad's face as he walked me down the aisle. And the look of happiness on his face as he handed me over to a man that he felt proud to call his son-in-law.

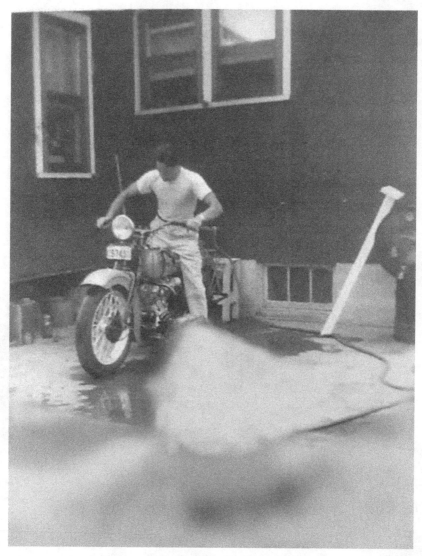

Dad on his Harley

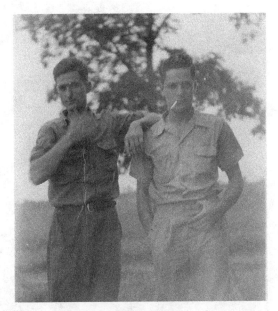

Uncle Joe and Dad on the farm

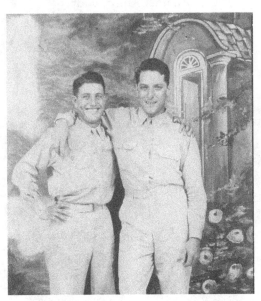

Dad (right) and his Army buddy in France, January 1945. This was the friend who was blown up next to him as they were running from enemy fire.

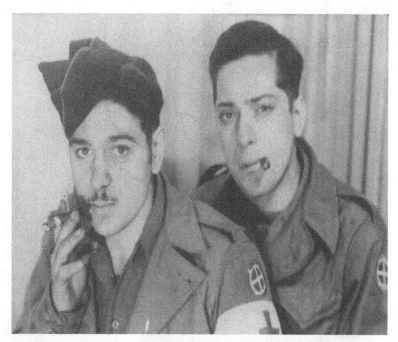

Another Army buddy

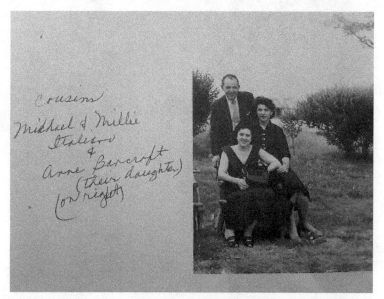

Cousins Millie and Mike Italiano and Anne Bancroft visiting Dad's farm.

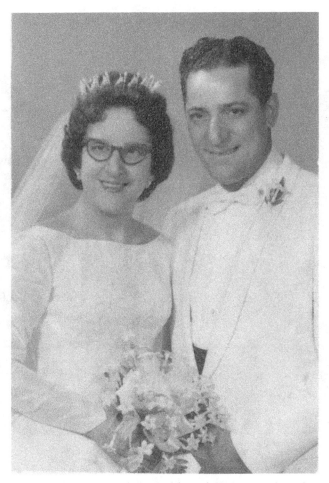

Mom and Dad on their wedding day, August 6, 1960

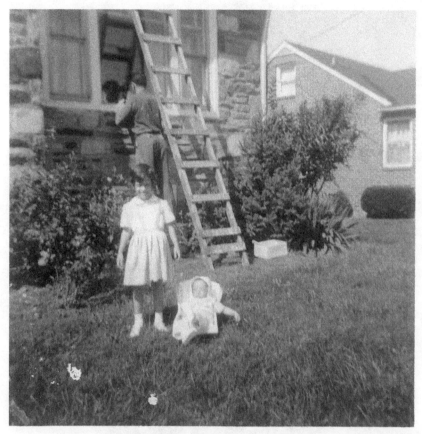

Always fixing something at our house

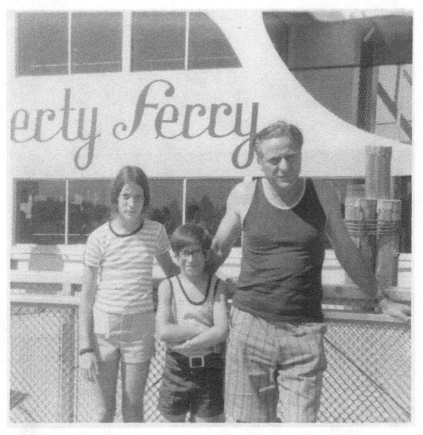

On one of our many day trips

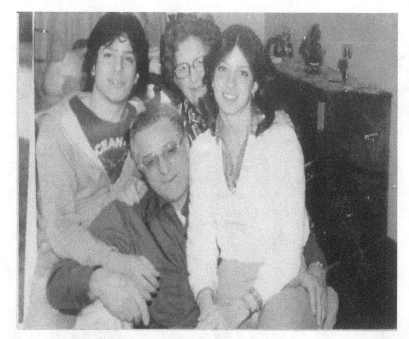

A loving family

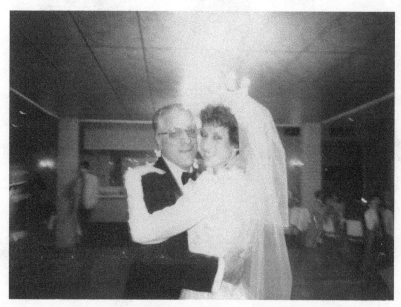

My wedding, November 16, 1985

CHAPTER 8

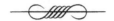

Now What Do We Do?

I had a good childhood…parents that loved me, a beautiful home, and financial security. However, we had a great deal of sickness in our extended family. My aunt, my mother's sister, was always very sickly and spent a significant amount of time in medical facilities. My mother's parents were also in poor health and in the hospital a majority of the time. My brother and I somewhat jokingly say that we grew up in hospital waiting rooms. But it is not too far from the truth. My mom and dad would visit whichever family member was sick at the time, and Sam and I would wait in the waiting room and do our homework. Sometimes, to entertain ourselves, we would ride up and down on the hospital elevators.

Along with our relative's ailments, our mother also had health issues. Because of the rheumatic fever she had as a child, she had some significant heart problems. However, she never let it stop her from being a wonderful mother and always doing so much for her family. As I said, she cooked, cleaned, grocery shopped, did the wash, ironed, helped with homework, and was the engine that made our family run.

As the years progressed, she started to show more severe signs of her heart issue. She would get out of breath very easily, and she became fatigued very quickly. But she kept pushing herself and never gave in to her limitations.

In the fall of 1985, about a month before my wedding in November, Mom had a mini stroke. She had been talking on the phone when her speech became slurred, and her mouth drooped. My dad noticed and immediately took her to the doctor.

After extensive testing, they determined that she had a blockage in her heart that needed to be removed before it led to another stroke that could potentially cause major damage. They wanted to immediately perform the surgery; however, my mother insisted that it needed to wait until after my wedding. The doctor acquiesced but said that it was imperative that it be done right after the wedding.

Jim and I were married on November 16, 1985. We left right afterward for our honeymoon, and Mom scheduled the surgery for the week that we came home. She went into the hospital on December 1 for what the doctor assured us was a minor procedure. My mother died on December 13, 1985.

The procedure did not go according to plan. We could never prove negligence, but in my heart, I felt that someone did not do what they were supposed to. The surgery apparently went fine, but afterward, she went into cardiac arrest, and it took an excessive amount of time to get her heart started again. When they did, she was left with brain damage and in a coma. She remained in a coma for over a week until I told her that it was okay for her to let go and that I would be fine. However, I lied. I did not know how I was ever going to be able to survive without her.

I had been a very overprotected, spoiled young woman up until this point in my life. I was not able to do anything without first consulting with Mom. She did everything for me. She did everything for all of us and took care of everyone. Dad, Sam, and I felt completely lost. We all looked at each other and thought the same thing... Now what do we do?

Somehow, we got through the funeral and Christmas that year. It's all a big blur when I think back on it now. But it was later, when everyone went home and back to their lives, that the horrible realization set in. We were like three lost ships in the ocean. Each of us was grieving in our own way, and we could not help each other. It was one of the most horrible times of my life.

I remember looking at my father, who was sixty-five at the time, and thinking that he would live the rest of his life alone. I remember thinking that he could live another twenty years, and he would be by himself. I was so incredibly sad for him.

I also realized that Dad did not know how to do many of the things that Mom had taken care of. Mom had always paid the bills and managed the financial aspects, so Dad had no idea what to do. I took him to the bank to find out how much money they had, and I had to show him how to write a check and pay bills. I also showed him how to do his wash and some basic housework. Our new life without Mom was so incredibly difficult for all of us.

After a few years and much therapy, I was able to enjoy life again. And my father got remarried. As much as I wanted him to be happy, it broke my heart to see him with someone else. Unfortunately, the woman he married was only after him for his money, and the marriage did not last long.

A few years later, Dad tried it again. This time, the woman was great. But they had come from two very different marriages previously. Dad was used to spending every minute with Mom, and that was what he was trying to replace. However, his new wife came from a marriage where she and her previous husband lived separate lives and only stayed together for the kids. So she was used to doing her own thing. Neither of them was getting what they wanted from this marriage. So, again, the marriage ended.

I think Dad realized, at this point, that he was trying to replace Mom, and that was not going to happen. He resigned himself to the fact that he was alone. This was difficult for him because he and Mom had had a great marriage, and he loved being married. I set out to help Dad find things to do.

He joined the YMCA and would go every day to work out. He loved to go for walks and went regularly regardless of the weather. He loved to garden, and he began to read extensively. He also began to go to New Jersey often to visit with his brothers Charlie and Joe. And Sam and I would visit and have him for dinner whenever we could.

When Jim's job took us to Albany, New York, for a promotion and a two-year rotation, I felt extreme guilt about leaving my father.

I cried and prayed about what to do. I moved kicking and screaming and with an ultimatum to my husband that I was coming back in two years with or without him. But in the end, we had a wonderful time living in New York, met great lifelong friends, and chose to stay for six years until Jim was transferred back to Pennsylvania. Dad came to see us often, and I went home to spend time with him as much as I could. And Sam was still nearby to help Dad and keep an eye on him.

Dad was doing fine on his own. He would cook for himself, clean, take care of his finances, and keep himself busy. Although he was alone, he seemed content. Just like all of us, he missed Mom every day. There was a huge hole in all of our hearts without her. But she had taught us to be strong and independent, and we all learned to survive without her—even Dad. She would have been very proud.

CHAPTER 9

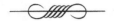

Pappers

My mother had dreamed of becoming a grandmother. She had loved being a mother and couldn't wait to nurture her future grandchildren. When Jim and I were talking about getting married, she talked about someday watching our children if I decided to go back to work. We had it all planned out. I would drop the kids off at Mom's on my way to work, along with any laundry that I needed done. She would watch the kids all day, do our laundry, and cook a meal for us, which I would take home and heat up for our dinner. I was spoiled, and I knew it. Life was going to be wonderful. Until Mom died, and nothing went according to our plan.

Dad, on the other hand, never talked about being a grandfather. While he was a terrific father, he was not overly affectionate. He had grown up in an unexpressive family where no one said "I love you" or outwardly showed their feelings. We knew that Dad loved us, but neither Sam nor I remember Dad telling us. His way of expressing his love was to provide for us and support us in whatever we wanted to do. We accepted that that was the way Dad showed affection. That was, until his grandchildren came along.

When our son Jimmy was born on July 3, 1990, Dad immediately showed up at the hospital. And the look of love on his face when he saw his grandson was beautiful. We had decided that Dad would be called "Grandpop" because that is what I had called my grandfather. As Jimmy grew up, he spent many hours bonding with his grandpop. And Dad was very affectionate with him, hugging and kissing him every chance he got, which came as a surprise to Sam and me. We often commented that we did not remember him being that way with us. But it was so special for me to observe.

Katelyn came along in 1994. Dad could not quite figure out what kind of name Katelyn was. He had grown up in a family of Marias, Theresas, Annas, and Angelinas. But her name did not matter. He instantly fell in love with her. She was his little "Katie Baby," as he affectionately started calling her. And the kids started calling Dad "Grandpappy." Over the years, Katelyn changed it to "Grandpappers" and then shortened it to "Pappers."

Dad idolized his grandchildren. He played in the yard with them, read to them, and held them when they were young. When they were little, he would sit and watch *Land Before Time* with Jimmy and *The Little Mermaid* with Katelyn repeatedly until he could practically recite them word for word. As they grew, he went to amusement parks, the beach, and on picnics with them.

When Katelyn was about seven, Dad and I had taken the kids to an amusement park. At that time, Dad was eighty-one years old. Katelyn spotted a ride in which you sat in a car shaped like a cow, and it whipped you around while the track the cow sat on also spun around. It was much like a Tilt-A-Whirl, only worse. Just watching it made my stomach turn. She looked at me hopefully and asked me to go on it with her. There was no way I could go on that ride without my lunch coming back up. So I told her no.

"Pappers, would you go on with me?" she asked her grandfather.

Without missing a beat, he grabbed her hand, and off they went to get in line for this barbaric ride. I watched in amazement as my eighty-one-year-old father was whipped and spun around while my daughter was laughing and thoroughly enjoying herself. When they got off, without anyone having regurgitated their food, Jimmy asked his grandfather to go on the roller coaster with him. And off they went.

As we arrived at the old, rickety, white roller coaster, I had some serious trepidations about my father going on this. This was not one of the new, smooth-riding roller coasters that many amusement parks had. This was an old, head-jostling, body-bashing one that I, at forty years old, was reluctant to get on. But Dad followed Jimmy into the line without a second thought. Again, I stood and watched in utter amazement as my elderly father got on this crazy, wild ride with his grandson. I remember telling the kids later that day to never expect me to do that with their kids when I was eighty-one years old!

Dad came to watch the kids sporting events, school plays, and anything that was important in their lives. When we had moved to Albany, New York, for six years for Jim's job, Dad drove for four hours to come see them. He was seventy-seven when we moved there and eighty-three when we moved back to Pennsylvania. He did this drive at least four times a year. I like to think he was coming to see me too, but I'm sure it was mostly to see the kids. Of course, we went to visit him also while we lived there because the kids loved seeing their Pappers.

Dad enjoyed coming to the beach with us in Ocean City, New Jersey. When the kids were young, he would sit in the sand and build sandcastles with them. As they got a little older, he would join them while they jumped in the waves. He even tried boogie boarding once or twice. And he loved going for long walks on the beach with both of them. But perhaps the most amazing activity that he would do with them was bike riding on the boardwalk. In his early eighties, he would gladly get on a bike and ride the whole length of the two and a half mile boardwalk with them and then turn around and ride back. He was eager and willing to do anything that the kids asked him to do.

It never ceased to amaze me how different Dad was with his grandchildren versus how he was with Sam and me. As I said, he was a wonderful father, but he was not overly affectionate with us. However, there was never a time that he was not hugging or kissing his grandchildren. And when Katelyn was younger, he was always holding her hand. I sometimes think he was making up for the fact that my children did not have their grandmother by giving them extra love. But mostly, I think he was just enjoying the wonderful grandchildren that he had been given, who loved their Pappers with all their hearts.

CHAPTER 10

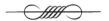

What the Heck Is Alzheimer's?

The first time I had heard of Alzheimer's disease was in 1985 when I was sitting in the waiting room at the hospital in Philadelphia, Pennsylvania, that my mother was being admitted to for her heart surgery. She and I were both reading magazines, and she looked up from the article that she was reading and exclaimed, "What a horrible disease!" She then proceeded to tell me about the article.

It stated that researchers were working to try to find a cure for Alzheimer's disease. It then went on to explain that Alzheimer's was an irreversible neurological disorder that slowly destroys memory and thinking skills and, eventually, the ability to perform the simplest tasks. Many times, the person progresses to the point of being incontinent, not recognizing their loved ones, and in need of constant care. The magazine article painted a horrendous picture of the disease and its progression.

After reading the article to me, Mom proclaimed, "How awful for not only the person with the disease but the caregiver. I hope I die before I ever get a disease like that." I had no way of knowing that Mom would get her wish. She never came home from the hospital.

Months after Mom died, when I was trying to find ways to cope with the terrible loss, I remembered what Mom had said. While I in no way was at peace with the fact that my mother died at sixty-three years old, I found a small amount of solace in the fact that she never lived long enough to develop this disease that she so feared. Little did I know that my father would be the unfortunate one.

No one that I knew had had Alzheimer's or knew anyone that had this debilitating disease. I do remember a distant relative when I was a young girl who asked me what my name was about twenty-five times while we were visiting on one occasion. But I remember the adults saying that he was senile. Being a young kid, I had no idea what that was other than maybe that was what happened when you got old. However, the only time that I had ever heard anything about Alzheimer's disease was when my mother had read that magazine article to me. So I had no idea what was happening when Dad started to exhibit some strange behaviors. However, over the years, I unfortunately learned a great deal about it.

When I lived in Albany, New York, I would call Dad every morning and every night. We would talk about what his plans were for the day or what he did that day, what the kids were doing, and how he was feeling. The conversations were not long, but I just wanted to check in with him. Sometimes he would tell me the same thing in our evening conversation that he had told me in the morning. I did not think this was a big deal because I sometimes repeated myself also.

However, over time, I started to notice that he would repeat the same thing in the same conversation. He would tell me in our nightly conversation that he went to New Jersey to visit his brother Joe that day and how my Uncle Joe was doing. Then a few minutes later, he would say, "Oh, I went to see Uncle Joe today."

I would respond with, "I know, Dad, you told me that."

And he would say, "Oh, that's right."

And we would laugh.

In another conversation, he would inquire about how the kids were doing. I would give him an update on how school was going and what activities they were involved in at that time. Then we would move on to what he had done that day. When that conversation was over, he would inquire about how the kids were doing again. I vacillated between being annoyed that he was not paying attention and being concerned about his memory.

Another questionable behavior that I noticed was his inability to find the right words. Sometimes we would be talking about something, and he would say a word that made no sense in the context of what we were discussing. Again, I wondered if he was just not concentrating on our conversation or if there was something more serious going on.

I started to see this repetition during our conversations and notice that he had trouble finding words more often. What was going on? Why was Dad repeating himself so much? Sam was noticing the same thing. Was this just normal aging? Should we bring it to his attention or just ignore it? Was this the first time we were seeing this behavior or had Dad exhibited this previously and we did not notice it? I began to reflect back on some of the strange incidents that had happened previously that had caused me to be concerned. And a feeling of dread started to present itself. Was Dad starting to exhibit signs of Alzheimer's disease? I decided to do some research.

CHAPTER 11

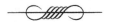

Early Glimpses

I learned in my research of Alzheimer's disease that the traits start to manifest themselves many years before the actual diagnosis. Alzheimer's can present as paranoia and agitation. There are little memory lapses and strange behaviors that loved ones may just chalk up to senior moments and normal aging. That was the case with Dad.

Looking back, there were signs many years before that we did not acknowledge. Or maybe we didn't want to acknowledge. One memory I have of a strange behavior happened years before Dad's diagnosis. He had been renting a house from a man named John that he knew from the YMCA that he belonged to. Dad had a portable phone at the time which, when it was not hung up on the charger, he kept on his coffee table.

He called me up one day, sounding very upset. He told me that he thought that John had been coming into the house when he was not there. I immediately got upset, thinking that he had stolen Dad's money or gone through his personal papers. I braced myself.

"How do you know this, Dad?" I asked him.

He responded, "Well, whenever I get off the phone, I put it face down on the coffee table, and when I came home today, it was face up."

I remember being both relieved and incredulous. Did he honestly think that John had come in and used his phone? I asked if anything else was out of place or missing, and he said no. When I asked if he could have just forgotten and put the phone down face up, he was adamant that he had not. We ended the conversation by agreeing that he should just keep an eye on things from then on and see if there was anything else that he noticed off-kilter.

We did not observe any other concerning behaviors while he was living there. However, a few years later, when he had moved into another house that he bought, there were some very strange incidents. In the kitchen of this house, behind a sliding closet door, there was a hot water heater. The heater could be turned off and on with a switch that resembled a light switch.

One morning, I received a phone call from Dad.

"Maryanne, I think someone broke into my house," Dad said as soon as I answered.

That feeling of dread again washed over me. "What happened, Dad? Why do you think that?" I asked.

He responded, "Well, I was trying to wash the dishes this morning, and there was no hot water. So I looked at the hot water heater switch, and it was turned off. Someone must have come in here and turned it off."

Once again, there was a feeling of relief but also shock that Dad actually thought that someone broke in and turned off his hot water heater. His TV was still there, money that he kept in his dresser was still there, and nothing else had been disturbed, except the switch for the hot water heater. Why would someone come in to just turn off his hot water heater?

Once again, I asked him if perhaps he mistakenly turned the switch off by accident, thinking it was the light switch, and again, he was adamant that he did not do it. I tried to reason with him and point out that if someone would have broken into his house, they would have taken his TV or money and done more than turn off the hot water heater. But there was no reasoning with him. These incidents became more frequent. And more bizarre.

After we had moved back to Pennsylvania from New York, I started noticing more and more concerning episodes happening with Dad since I was seeing him more often now. Not only was he repeating himself and exhibiting some paranoia, but I also started noticing that he was misplacing many items and putting them in strange places. On one occasion, Dad could not find his pillbox. He told me he had looked everywhere for it but could not locate it. I went to his house and began searching high and low for it. I looked in drawers, in the sofa cushions, in the trash can, anywhere that I thought Dad could have accidentally placed it. It was nowhere to be found.

So I went out and bought him another pillbox and filled it with his weekly pills. I placed it on the kitchen counter where his other one was always kept. Months went by with no other occurrences of a missing pillbox.

One day, I was trying to find an umbrella in Dad's closet for him to use when we went out that day. There was not an umbrella on the floor of the closet, so I reached up to the top shelf, which I had to stand on my toes to reach, and lo and behold, there was Dad's old pillbox.

When I called Dad over to show him what I had found, he said, "How the hell did that get there?"

I asked him if he had put it there, and he insisted that he did not. Rather than upset him, I let it go.

Many items in Dad's house started showing up in strange places. The TV remote was in his car, a screwdriver was in the washing machine, and medicine boxes were tacked up on the wall in his kitchen. His hat and coat were hung on a sconce in the living room instead of in his coat closet. Again, rather than upset or embarrass him, I would just move the items to a more "normal" location.

One day, Dad called me in a panic because he could not find his wallet. Because I knew that Dad's two prized possessions were his watch and his wallet, I realized how upset this was most likely making him. I raced to his house, and we began the search.

I called Sam to see if he had seen it. In one of those "if you don't laugh, you'll cry" moments, he suggested that I look in the refrigerator. After we laughed about it, I did, in fact, look in the refrigerator. It wasn't there.

After our extensive search, I broke the bad news to Dad that, since we could not find his wallet, we were going to have to replace it. He was very upset about losing his license. At this point, we were starting to question whether Dad should be driving anymore, but neither Sam nor I wanted to be the one to have to take his license away.

I assured Dad that we would get the license replaced. We went out and bought a new wallet, and I proceeded to call about all the replacement cards that he needed—his Veterans Administration card, his Medicare card, prescription cards, etc. Sam took him to get his license replaced. Within a week, he had all his new cards in his new wallet, and Dad was happy again. Life was good—he had his watch and his wallet.

About a month later, Dad and I were getting ready to head out for one of our walks. Since it was cold outside, I suggested that he wear his gloves and hat. He reached into the drawer in his dresser and pulled out a hat that I had not seen him wear in a very long time. As he went to put it on, something fell out and landed on his head. It was his old wallet. And, once again, he asked his infamous question, "How the hell did that get there?" Rather than ask him if he put it there, which I knew he would deny, I just took it from him and brought it home with me to put in a safe place. I had a feeling we were going to need a replacement wallet again in the near future.

What was going on with Dad? What was causing him to do these strange things? How was he not able to remember turning off his hot water heater? Why was he placing these items in odd places? Why was he repeating himself so much? Was he just getting old and forgetful? Or was it something worse? Was it Alzheimer's disease?

CHAPTER 12

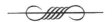

Home Improvements

Dad was very meticulous whenever he repaired or remodeled anything in his house. And as I said previously, he could repair anything. However, in hindsight, as his disease progressed, there were things that he did that made us scratch our heads.

On one occasion, he had decided to paint the front porch on his house. It was a concrete slab that had been painted a slate gray color previously. The paint had started to chip, so Dad felt that he should repaint it. We asked him if he needed help, but he was very independent, and he insisted that he could to do it himself.

A few days later, Dad had finished the job. I couldn't wait to see the finished product. As I was pulling into Dad's driveway, I noticed a glow coming from the front of his house. As I got closer, I found out where the glow was coming from. Dad had painted the porch a glossy neon purple! It was literally radiating. I was astounded that he had actually picked that color. Not only had he picked a ridiculous color, but he had also gotten paint all over the white siding.

Dad had painted his whole life—rooms in the farmhouse that he grew up in, rooms in my childhood home, the outside of our house, etc. Each time he painted, the job was meticulously done, with not a drop of paint on anything else but the object that he was painting. So seeing purple paint splattered on the white siding was shocking, to say the least. Obviously, he did not see the same thing that I saw because he was very proud of how his new porch looked. Not wanting to burst his bubble, I told him it looked great. Then I prepared Sam for what he would see the next time that he visited Dad.

A few weeks later, Dad decided to paint the deck in his backyard. He went out to buy paint and got to work. He called me a few days later and told me that he had completed the painting job, and he could not wait to show me his beautiful back deck.

On my next visit, I cautiously walked around to Dad's backyard. And I was greeted with his new orange deck! It had been a beautiful walnut color previously, and now it was a bright orange. Was Dad buying the discounted paint at the hardware store that no one else wanted?

He was so proud of the job that he had done that I did not have the heart to tell him what I really thought. So I smiled and told him that it looked great while inside I was thinking, *Oh my god, how can we repaint this without him knowing?* Dad's judgment was obviously starting to suffer.

Around this same time, my husband and I were doing some renovations at our house. Since I had always asked Dad for help whenever we were doing any home improvement projects, I asked him to come over and help us put a new showerhead in. He immediately agreed to help since he was always more than happy to assist with anything Sam or I ever needed.

Dad came to our house with his toolbox and listened while we told him what we needed him to do. Off he went to our upstairs bathroom to install our new showerhead. In the meantime, Jim and I were working in our kitchen, installing crown molding around the ceiling. Our kitchen was directly underneath the bathroom that Dad was working in.

As I was on the ladder working on the molding, I started to notice water dripping from the ceiling. I thought I was seeing things at first. But as I kept looking, the dripping became more intense. At about this same time, I heard Dad shouting from upstairs. I jumped off the ladder and ran upstairs to find him trying desperately to stem the flow of water coming from the pipe coming out of the wall. He had apparently forgotten to turn off the water at the main valve before taking the old showerhead off.

I immediately ran down two flights of steps to the main water valve to shut off the water. Then I went back to the kitchen to start cleaning up the water that had dripped through the ceiling from the bathroom. In the meantime, Dad was pretty shaken up. He felt so bad for the damage that he had caused. While I was upset about the leak, I was more incredulous about the fact that my father, who had done extensive plumbing work in our house when I was growing up and was very knowledgeable about anything plumbing related, had forgotten something as simple as shutting the main water valve off.

We had decided that in the future we would give Dad easier jobs to do in which there would be no danger of him making such a significant mistake. So the next time Dad came to visit, I asked him if he could put up our new vertical blinds on our sliding glass door. As always, he was more than happy to help. He got out his toolbox and went to work with his power drill and screws. When the job was complete, our vertical blinds looked beautiful.

I thanked Dad for his help and complimented him on the terrific job that he had done. I made dinner for all of us, and then Dad left for home. Later that evening, when darkness came, I went over to shut the vertical blinds. As I pulled the cord to move the blinds, the entire mechanism came crashing to the floor!

Jim got up on a ladder to look to see what had happened. Apparently, Dad had used one-inch screws and screwed them into the drywall instead of using two-and-a-half-inch screws and screwing them into the studs. Even in my limited knowledge about construction, I knew that you should not screw into drywall with such small screws and expect them to hold up the weight of the vertical blinds.

How had Dad not known this? I can not emphasize enough the fact that he could build, fix, repair, install just about anything that needed to be built, fixed, repaired, or installed. So how did he not know that such small screws installed into drywall would not hold all that weight?

From the research that I had done so far, Dad was very obviously exhibiting the many signs of Alzheimer's disease. His lack of judgment, paranoia, constant repetition, forgetfulness, and strange behaviors were all pointing to this dreaded disease. It was definitely time to see his doctor and get a professional opinion.

CHAPTER 13

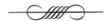

Realization Setting In

In the fall of 2005, we had decided to take Dad to a neurologist to have him evaluated. It was becoming very obvious that his memory was declining, his judgment was off, and he was not the father that we knew. He was diagnosed with the early stages of Alzheimer's disease.

Dad was confused about what this meant. And I only had a limited knowledge of what Alzheimer's was or what it entailed. The doctor explained it to us as best as he could and told us that there presently was no cure for the disease. He explained that the disease affects people differently and that it progresses at different rates for everyone. It felt like a death sentence, and I tried not to let Dad see how upset this news had made me.

The doctor told us that there were some medications that could slow the progression of the disease. Apparently, people had been seeing some positive results from them. So Dad agreed to try the first of many that he would eventually try.

A week after Dad started his new medication, my family was going away on a week-long vacation. I was very worried about leaving Dad alone, but Sam assured me that he would keep an eye on him and make sure everything was okay. I called Dad every day to check in, and he seemed fine during all of our phone conversations.

One night, I decided to call Sam and see how things were going. The conversation was very stilted. When I asked him how Dad was doing, Sam was very elusive and told me to have a good time, and we would have a discussion when I arrived home. I had to choose between ruining my family's vacation and pressuring Sam to tell me what was going on or to just let Sam handle whatever was happening and try to enjoy myself. I chose the latter.

As soon as I got home, I received the story from Sam. Dad had called him one night and said that he needed him to come over. When Sam arrived at Dad's, he was walking around the house with his gun, which thankfully wasn't loaded. But he told Sam that he had heard something and insisted that there was an intruder in his house. Sam proceeded to turn the house upside down, looking in every closet, under every bed, and in the attic until Dad was convinced that there was no one in the house. Sam went to the hardware store to buy new locks and deadbolts and then installed them on all the doors. Dad felt much better. But he was experiencing extreme paranoia.

I called his doctor immediately to tell him what had happened. He told me that one in one thousand people suffer from paranoia from the Alzheimer's medication that Dad had been placed on. It seems that Dad was that one person. So he promptly took him off of it.

Over the course of Dad's battle with Alzheimer's disease, his doctor tried many other medications in the hopes of slowing the progression of the disease. Unfortunately, we did not think at the time that they were helping. In hindsight, perhaps they did help because he declined slowly over an eight-year period. But at the time, we were hoping for a miracle pill that would bring our father back.

One of the medications that Dad was using was in the form of a patch. He was supposed to place the patch on his chest or stomach in the morning and then remove it the next morning and affix another one. I called him every morning to walk him through this routine. Our conversations went something like this, "Okay, Dad, unbutton your shirt and pull off the patch that is on your chest." After he told me that he did it, I would then say, "Now open a new packet, pull out the patch and put it on your chest." He would put the phone down, and I could hear him rip open the packet and move around following my directions. This conversation would be repeated every day.

A month into this routine, Dad had to visit his cardiologist for a checkup. I would accompany him into the examination room for these visits because he would only have to remove his shirt so there was no risk of Dad losing his dignity. I also wanted to be there to answer any questions that he might not understand, as information was getting harder for him to process.

Once the nurse got Dad settled in the exam room, she explained that she was going to attach electrodes to his chest so that she could do an EKG. She asked him to remove his shirt. As Dad proceeded to unbutton his shirt, a patch became visible on his chest. As he undid another button, another patch became visible. Another button, another patch. As he removed his shirt, I began to count the patches. There were ten! Apparently, Dad had not been removing the old ones when he was applying the new ones. I was horrified.

The nurse and I began to peel all of them off of Dad without bringing his attention to it. She and I looked at each other in shock and amazement. So many thoughts were going through my head. Why was he not removing the old patches? Were my directions not clear enough? What damage was being done to him by having so many of them on? The nurse could see my obvious concern and alarm and quickly went to get the doctor.

The cardiologist came into the room fifteen minutes later and told me that he looked up information on the patch and that each one was a 4.6 milligram daily dose that was absorbed by his body. While the instructions say to remove the old one before applying the new one, the doctor felt that once the dosage was absorbed, the old patch did not present any danger to Dad. He reassured me that I did not need to worry about it.

Even with the doctor's assurance that Dad was fine, I still felt awful. I realized that he was no longer able to follow multistep directions. This realization was going to change many of the ways that we were caring for him.

As the cardiologist finished his examination of Dad, another realization occurred to me. The doctor told me that Dad's heart was in terrific shape, and that he was in better shape than many sixty-year-old men that he saw. While this was wonderful news, it was also a double-edged sword. This meant that physically, Dad could live a very long time while mentally he would progressively decline. I left the doctor's office that day with a sense of doom. I also decided to do more research so that I could be prepared for what was to come.

CHAPTER 14

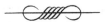

Alzheimer's Facts and Figures

While I usually find research to be helpful in times of fear of the unknown, in the case of Dad's diagnosis, the facts were devastating. But I felt that I needed to know as much as I could about this disease and what it would mean for our family. So I set out to learn the facts and figures of Alzheimer's disease.

Alzheimer's disease is named after the German physician Alois Alzheimer. In 1901, Dr. Alzheimer examined a fifty-one-year-old patient named Auguste Deter in Frankfurt Hospital in Germany. The woman had been experiencing problems with memory and language, as well as various psychological problems, such as disorientation and hallucinations. When Dr. Alzheimer examined her, she was sitting in her hospital bed with a confused, helpless expression on her face. When Dr. Alzheimer asked her what her name was, she replied, "Auguste." Next, he asked her what her last name was, and she replied, "Auguste." When he asked her what her husband's name was, she replied, "Auguste." As she was answering these questions, she was eating her lunch of cauliflower and pork. When Dr. Alzheimer asked her what she was eating, she replied, "Spinach."

Dr. Alzheimer noted Deter's impaired comprehension, memory, and judgment, as well as her paranoia and disorientation. She did not know what year it was, was unable to write her name, or perform basic math. At this time, there was no term to describe this condition. The symptoms were much like senility that affected the elderly, but this woman was middle aged. How could she have symptoms of senility at her age?

When Deter died in 1906, Dr. Alzheimer autopsied her brain. He found that her brain was roughly half the size of a normal, healthy one. He also found neurofibrillary tangles that wrapped around the interior of the cells, crushing them. Along with these tangles, he found amyloid plaques. These tangles and plaques would be the hallmark of Alzheimer's disease as scientists know it today. A few years after Deter had died and Dr. Alzheimer had presented his findings at psychoanalytical lectures, it was proposed by his boss that the disease be named after him.

Every sixty-six seconds, someone in the United States develops Alzheimer's disease. There are over five million Americans living with Alzheimer's today, and by the year 2050, that number is projected to rise to fourteen million, barring the development of medical breakthroughs to prevent, slow, or cure the disease. While deaths from other major causes have decreased, records indicate that deaths from Alzheimer's disease have increased significantly. Between 2000 and 2018, deaths from Alzheimer's disease increased 146 percent while deaths from heart disease, the number one cause of death, have decreased 7.8 percent. Alzheimer's is the sixth leading cause of death in the United States and the fifth leading cause of death among those sixty-five and older. One in three seniors dies from Alzheimer's. It kills more than breast cancer and prostate cancer combined. People age sixty-five and older survive an average of four to eight years after a diagnosis of Alzheimer's, yet some live as long as twenty years with the disease. Among people age seventy, 61 percent of those with Alzheimer's are expected to die before the age of eighty compared with 30 percent of people without Alzheimer's.

There are five stages to the disease. Someone in the first stage does not show any overt signs or symptoms related to thinking or reasoning, according to Verna R. Porter, MD, neurologist and director of the Alzheimer's Disease Program at Providence Saint John's Health Center in Santa Monica, California. The patient appears or feels normal and healthy, but there are internal and metabolic changes happening in the body that will only appear in medical testing.

In the second stage, the memory loss symptoms could sometimes be confused with that of a normal aging adult. The person may experience confusion and some memory loss, but they will still have the ability to make decisions and engage in conversation.

The third stage is where the most common symptoms of the disease appear—clear, persistent, memory loss and challenges with problem-solving. Patients in this stage will need help with handling finances, managing medication, shopping for groceries, and meal preparation, to a name a few. These activities are called instrumental activities of daily living or IADLs. These are actions that are important to being able to live independently but are not necessarily required activities on a daily basis. Patients will try to compensate for their memory loss or confusion and still try to perform these functions, but in most cases, will have difficulty. This is the time for family members or caregivers to schedule a meeting with a physician to discuss the diagnosis and plans for the future.

In stage four of the disease, your loved one might wander, not remember who you are or how to care for themselves. They have little to no independent functioning and can only do simple chores. Driving is unsafe at this stage. There is more profound memory loss at this point along with mood or behavior changes. The patient may get very agitated and suspicious, and they should not be left alone at this stage. In some cases, there will be a change in the patient's personality, and they may become combative and angry at those around them.

During the last stage of Alzheimer's disease, the patient has severe memory loss and can no longer judge time or place. In this stage, the patient is no longer able to perform activities of daily living or ADLs. These activities include the following: caring for their personal hygiene, being able to dress and undress themselves, being able to feed themselves, maintaining continence, and transferring, which is the ability to move oneself from a seated to standing position or to get into and out of bed. The patient may also no longer be able to walk or talk. In this stage of the disease, the patient will require help with all these activities and will be fully reliant on their caregivers. At this point, it is time to discuss hospice care and making the patient as comfortable as possible.

One symptom that can occur during any stage of the disease, but tends to peak in the middle stages, is a behavior called sundowning. When someone becomes confused, anxious, aggressive, or restless consistently in late afternoon or early evening, it is called sundowning. It is also known as "late-day confusion." It is thought to be a problem for 66 percent of people with Alzheimer's and can severely affect their quality of life. Some of the causes are the following: being tired at the end of the day, disruption of the circadian cycle (sleep/wake pattern) due to Alzheimer's, consuming a large meal at the end of the day, especially if they consume caffeine or alcohol, and low lighting and increased shadows which causes the patient to misinterpret what they see and become confused.

To help a loved one experiencing sundowning, it is important to have them stick to the same schedule every day. It is also helpful to keep their home well lit in the evening with some studies suggesting light therapy to reduce agitation and confusion. Avoiding any types of stimulants, such as caffeine, alcohol, or nicotine is also helpful, as well as keeping their evening meal modest. At this stage of the disease, watching television or reading a book might be too difficult for them in the evening and may cause added stress and frustration. Instead, consider playing soft music to create a calm and quiet environment. Try to fill their home and surroundings with things they find familiar and comforting. Keeping track of what triggers the sundowning in your loved one will help you to avoid the situations that promote agitation and confusion.

Over the years of dealing with Dad's illness, I became a wealth of knowledge on the subject of Alzheimer's disease. I found myself researching anything that I could get my hands on to become as educated as possible about it, as well as the stages and symptoms that are characteristic of the disease. I learned of numerous ways in which to assist Dad in coping with the many changes that were occurring.

I also found myself constantly looking for any medical breakthroughs that might help to combat the disease. Unfortunately, over the eight years of Dad's battle with Alzheimer's, the statistics got worse, and there were no medical miracles. No single drug had yet been approved that had been shown to slow the progress of this devastating neurodegenerative disease. The future did not look bright for us.

CHAPTER 15

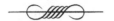

The Game Plan

After Dad's diagnosis, Sam and I had put a game plan together to care for him. I would go to Dad's house every Sunday to clean, do his wash, fill up his pillbox for the week, and just check up on him. I would also visit one night during the week after work. Sam's day was Tuesday, his day off. He would take Dad to any doctor appointments he had and do his grocery shopping with him. He would also try to visit one night during the week.

Dad was still driving at this point, so he would go for a walk at a nearby park every day to get some exercise. However, he knew that he was slipping mentally and did not trust himself to travel much more than that on his own. So he waited for Sam or me to drive him to places outside his comfort zone.

One area in which we noticed a significant decline was in the area of Dad's hygiene. Dad had always been fastidious about his appearance. When I was growing up, I remember him taking a longer time in the bathroom than my mother. He would take a long shower, put on deodorant, comb every hair in place, and come out looking meticulous. He had always taken great pride in how he looked. That all changed as his Alzheimer's disease progressed.

Many times, when I would get to Dad's house, he would smell of body odor. He would have spent the past few days working in the yard and sweating but would have neglected to take a shower. When I would ask him if he was still showering regularly, he would insist that he was. But by the stench of him, he obviously was not. I knew that Dad was starting to have some balance issues at the time also, so I wondered if he was frightened of getting in the shower and falling. I struggled with trying not to embarrass Dad by telling him that he did not smell clean. So I gently suggested that he take a shower while I was there in case he lost his balance and fell in the shower. I assured him I would not come in if I heard him fall, but that, at least, I would be there if he had a problem and could call for help. He liked this idea and started to take his showers whenever Sam and I would visit.

I also noticed that he was neglecting to put his dirty clothes in the clothes hamper. I would get ready to do his laundry, and there would be no clothes in the hamper from the prior week when I had done his wash. I decided to investigate by looking in his closet. As I opened his closet door, I was greeted by the foul odor of unwashed shirts. He had been hanging up his sweaty shirts after taking them off. Again, not wanting to embarrass him, my new game plan each time I went to visit was to go into his closet and smell his shirts. Whichever shirts smelled unclean were pulled out and thrown in the washing machine.

His hair was another issue. For a man who had always spent a significant amount of time making sure every hair was in place, it was hard to see him with his hair unruly and uncombed. Dad had a full head of beautiful silver hair, but many times when I would go to visit him, he resembled Albert Einstein with his hair sticking up in all directions. I would encourage him to go into the bathroom and fix his hair before we went out for our trip to the store or for a walk, which he would do reluctantly. As meticulous as Dad had been with his appearance, he had also been that way about his home. He had always made sure everything was clean and neat. Like his appearance, he took great pride in how his home looked. That was before Alzheimer's disease.

Many times, when I would get there on Sundays, I would have to thoroughly clean his bathroom as he had obviously had some toileting issues and had neglected to clean up after himself. So as not to embarrass Dad, I would tell him that I had to go to the bathroom.

He must have thought I had some serious stomach issues as I would be in there for quite some time cleaning.

When Sam would go visit with Dad, he would help him take care of the outside of the house. Dad was still cutting his own grass at this time. However, like his house, his lawn was starting to suffer. Dad's yard used to look impeccable, with the lines perfectly parallel and every blade of grass cut uniformly. However, now there were huge patches of grass that were not cut, and the lines were going every which way. We had told him that we wanted to get someone to come and cut his grass for him, but he was adamant about doing it himself. So, many times, Sam would tell Dad that he wanted the exercise and cut the grass for him.

Paying his bills and taking care of his finances was another area of concern. After Mom died, Dad had to learn how to do this since it was something that Mom had always taken care of. So he developed a very organized system of putting any bills that needed to be paid in a Pendaflex folder marked "To Be Paid." He would check the folder periodically, and once he paid a bill, move the stub, on which he wrote "Paid" to another Pendaflex folder marked "Paid Bills." He never missed paying a bill in all the years that he did this. He also balanced his checkbook to the penny every month.

As his memory declined more and more, I began checking his "To Be Paid" folder. I found bills that had been due months earlier and a few "Late Notices" along with the original bill. I also found bills to be paid in the "Paid" folder. And then there was his electric bill that was paid three times. And there was no rhyme or reason to his checkbook. There were deposits that were deducted and withdrawals that were added. It was time for me to take over Dad's finances.

We were walking a fine line between taking over many of Dad's jobs and still trying to have him retain some independence. On one occasion, when we suggested doing something for him, he said, "You're taking everything away from me." He was a very proud man, and we did not want to make him feel incompetent in any way. So it became very tricky at times.

Over time, we were able to convince Dad that Sam and I were just trying to relieve him of some of these burdens that were mundane and that it was not that we didn't think he could handle them. We were just helping him so that he could have more time to do the things he enjoyed, like going for walks and reading. He seemed to fall for it because he readily turned over some of these chores to us. And some of the jobs that we took over were done stealthily, so he seemed to be happy with the arrangement. Sam and I worked as a team and were able to manage all these new undertakings that we had to take on. However, as the disease progressed, we were starting to get overwhelmed.

We felt that, for the most part, our game plan was going well. We were able to care for Dad's physical needs and handle many of his other responsibilities. However, we felt that Dad needed more care and companionship at this point, and Sam and I could not juggle anymore. Between working and caring for our own needs, as well as Dad's, we could no longer do this on our own. So it was time to bring in reinforcements.

CHAPTER 16

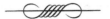

Barbara

It was quickly becoming obvious that we had to put more procedures in place to care for Dad. His doctor did not feel that he needed constant care yet. We just needed to check on him more often than the visits that Sam and I were already doing. Along came an angel sent by God.

Due to the fact that Sam and I both worked, we knew that we could not get there during the day. We thought that if we could get someone to come in two to three afternoons a week to just visit with Dad and be our eyes and ears, that would greatly help our situation. So I contacted a home health agency that Dad just happened to have a brochure for lying on his coffee table. When I asked him where he got the brochure, he had no idea. Divine intervention? One of the many that we experienced over the course of Dad's long illness.

When I called the agency and told them what I was looking for and the type of nurturing, patient person that would be the best fit for Dad, they immediately recommended a woman named Barbara. They told me that she had just started with them but that she was a warm, wonderful person who thoroughly enjoyed working with the elderly. We made arrangements to meet her at a restaurant the following week so that I could see for myself if she would be a good candidate. I was going to go with a mental checklist of what we were looking for.

There are times in your life where you meet someone that you have an immediate connection and kinship with. That is what happened with Barbara. When I introduced her to Dad, she went right up to him and hugged him. A check mark was placed on my mental checklist next to the word "nurturing."

We all sat down and began to talk. I explained to Barbara that we wanted someone to come in a few hours two to three days a week to just check on Dad and keep him company. Even though I had explained this to Dad before we went to meet Barbara, he said, "Oh, I don't need anyone to do that. I'm fine." Barbara immediately jumped in and said, "Well, I hear you love to go for walks, Sam, so I was thinking maybe you and I could just go for walks together. I love to walk too, and I don't like to go alone."

Bingo! Dad's face lit up, and he said, "Oh, I'd like that. That sounds great!" Check marks were placed next to "brilliant," "clever," and "thoughtful" on my checklist. She had realized that Dad was trying to appear independent, and she found a way to let him keep his dignity.

The rest of the evening went pretty much the same, with me placing mental check marks down my entire list of requirements. She was incredible. And I could tell that Dad loved her. She was ready to start whenever we needed her.

I called the agency the next day, and Barbara started coming to Dad's house every Monday, Wednesday, and Friday from 12:00 p.m. to 3:00 p.m. They went for long walks at all of Dad's favorite parks. They would sit and have long conversations. Sometimes they would stop and get a soda or a milkshake. She always left me detailed notes about what they did and what they talked about. I got the impression from her heartfelt notes that she enjoyed their afternoons together just as much as Dad did.

Dad would get so excited when, during my morning phone call to him, I would tell him that Barbara was coming that day. He would say, "She's such a wonderful girl." Barbara was in her fifties at the time, so she and I would get such a chuckle out of him calling her a "girl." Dad truly loved Barbara.

And, likewise, so did Sam and I. She became a member of our family. To this day, I do not think she truly knows what a godsend she was. During Dad's illness, I was working, caring for two teenagers, taking care of all Dad's financial and medical needs, and, for some of that time, caring for Jim, who had had a spinal cord injury in 2009 that left him partially paralyzed. I was literally spent physically and emotionally. Barbara gave me the peace of mind that I needed to know that Dad was in good hands when she was there. As I said, she was an angel sent by God.

Barbara had decided to leave the agency that she was with so that she could pursue other interests. When she told me this, my heart sank. However, she then told me that she had grown to love Dad and that she hoped she could still spend time with him. I was elated.

She continued to see Dad three times a week for many years after that. Her visits then started to include taking him to some of his many doctor appointments and then, eventually, visiting him in his assisted-living facility when he needed more care.

Barbara was with Dad up until the very end. She and I would cry on the phone together when we would discuss how painful it was to watch him decline. He could not remember her name at the end, but he still smiled when she walked in, and he still said, "Hi, sweetheart" when he saw her.

On the day that Dad died, the first person I called to tell was my son, who was away at school. The next person was Barbara. She was his second daughter. She asked if she could come over to see him. I told her Dad would want that.

When she got there twenty minutes later, she sat next to Dad's body and held his hand. With tears streaming down her face, she told him that she loved him and that she would always remember their special times together. Dad was truly a lucky man to have had Barbara in his life.

Dad's funeral was private. Sam and I did not have the energy to be social or put together an elaborate send-off. And Dad would not have wanted that. He was a simple man. So his family all stood by his casket and read letters that we had written to him and kissed him goodbye. He was surrounded by the people who loved him and whom he truly loved and who meant the world to him—myself, Sam, Jim, Jimmy, and Katelyn.

And Barbara!

CHAPTER 17

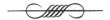

Unable to Learn Something New

As we started noticing more and more strange behaviors that Dad was exhibiting, we became increasingly concerned. His memory loss, poor judgment, and paranoia were obvious signs of his diagnosis. However, one area of his decline shocked me. This was his inability to learn anything new.

I had grown up watching this intelligent man be able to figure out how to put things together without reading the instructions or how to fix anything that was broken. He could learn anything that he put his mind to. So I had a difficult time understanding how he had lost this ability.

Sam and I had decided to get Dad a cell phone so that he could always have it with him when he went out. We felt better knowing that if he had any issues, he could call for help immediately. It never occurred to me that he would not be able to learn how to use it.

I found a cell phone that was very basic and easy to use since Dad had never owned a cell phone before. It had an on and off button and a keypad. Dad would be able to use this with no problem. Or so I thought.

I explained to him exactly what he needed to do. I told him that, unlike his portable phone in which you dialed the number and the call went right through, with a cell phone, you have to press "send" after dialing the number. We practiced a number of times, and he seemed to have gotten it. At least, I thought he did.

Apparently, according to him, he had tried to call me a number of times on his new phone the next day, and I never answered. However, I had not received a single call from him. He insisted that he called me but that I had not picked up the phone. When I asked him if he had pushed the "send" button after he dialed my number, he could not remember. I had a feeling that he had not, and that is why the call did not go through.

We worked on the cell phone instructions repeatedly for the next few weeks. We went over it and over it, and Dad could not learn how to use it. Or if he did, he could not retain what he had learned. Rather than cause him aggravation and frustration, we decided to abandon the cell phone idea. However, that was not the only gadget that Dad could not master.

We had decided to have an alarm installed in his house so that he would feel safer, and we would feel more at peace. After the alarm company installed it, they explained the simple instructions to Dad. All that he had to do was push the "ON" button to turn the alarm on and the "OFF" button to turn it off. The tricky part was when he was leaving the house. Then he was to push a different button that had a timer. After pushing the button, he had thirty seconds to open the door, go out, and close it behind him. If he did not do this in thirty seconds, a signal would be sent to the alarm company, and they would call Dad's house, and he would have to give them a password. If he did not answer or was unable to give them the correct password, the police would be sent.

You can imagine how this went. There were times that he pushed the button with the timer, and then instead of leaving the house, he decided to go to the bathroom first. Or he pushed the button and then decided to read the newspaper instead of going out. Each time, the alarm company would call, and Dad would have to recite the password. Interestingly, even though his memory was declining, he always remembered the password, which was Mary, my mother's name.

After numerous times of having the alarm company call to check in, they began to become concerned and called me to suggest that this may not be working for him. As much as I did not want to admit it, they were right. Dad was unable to remember the steps necessary to activate the alarm. Unfortunately, we had to have it disconnected.

As I began to realize that Dad no longer had the ability to learn anything new, I feared that the everyday creature comforts that he was so used to would break and need to be replaced. This would mean that he would have to learn how to use new items. His automatic coffee maker, his garage door opener, and his portable phone were just a few of the things that he used every day that I prayed would not become inoperable and need to be replaced. For someone who relied on his morning coffee each morning, how would he ever be able to learn how to use a new coffee maker if we could not find an identical one to replace his? And how would he ever learn to use a new portable phone if his present one died? It was a constant concern as Dad's disease progressed.

CHAPTER 18

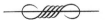

Mini Mental Exam

As Dad was moving through the stages of Alzheimer's disease, Sam and I had to take on many additional responsibilities and handle many more of his activities of daily living. Bill paying, cleaning, grocery shopping, grass cutting all became too much for Dad to handle. So Sam and I shared these chores.

Doctor's visits also became something that Dad could no longer do on his own. He showed up for one of his doctor's appointments a week early even though he had the reminder card, with the date and time, right on his kitchen counter where he could clearly see it. Another time he went to his dentist appointment and told his dentist about the gout that he was suffering from in his foot and asked him to prescribe medication for it. The dentist called me after Dad's appointment to suggest that my brother or I come to his next dental cleaning.

As Dad aged, there were more and more doctor appointments—cardiologists, neurologists, rheumatologists, audiologists, dermatologists, ophthalmologists, urologists, podiatrists, etc. The "ists" were endless. Each doctor appointment was upsetting in its own way. Each appointment brought home the fact that Dad was aging and many systems were starting to fail.

Perhaps the most upsetting of these numerous appointments was with his neurologist who gave Dad a test to check the progression of his Alzheimer's disease. We needed to know where he was on the scale that ranked the disease from mild to severe in order to plan for his future care. The test that his doctor administered was called the MMSE or Mini-Mental State Exam. This is a test that is given to measure cognitive impairment in people with Alzheimer's disease. The test is a thirty-point questionnaire that tests orientation to time and place, recall, comprehension, cognition, and function.

When the doctor started to administer the test, he asked me if I would like to stay. I thought this was a strange question because I had taken Dad to the appointment, so why wouldn't I want to stay? It quickly became apparent why the doctor thought I might not want to be in the room.

The first question the doctor asked Dad was, "What is your name?"

Dad very confidently answered, "Sam."

Next was, "Do you know where you are today?"

Dad chuckled and said, "Yes, I'm in a doctor's office."

So far, so good. I was so proud that he was getting all the answers correct. Then it slowly started to go awry.

"Sam, do you know where you live?" asked the doctor.

"Yes," Dad replied. "In New Jersey." He lived in Pennsylvania.

I started to explain to the doctor that he grew up in New Jersey, so that was an honest mistake, but the doctor quickly silenced me with a shake of his head. Okay, I thought, it is only one question. Next, he asked Dad how old he was.

Dad replied, "Sixty-five."

He was eighty-eight at the time. Next came, "What season is it?"

Dad replied, "Winter."

It was spring. I was quickly becoming concerned.

At the time of this MMSE, it was 2008, and George Bush was the president. The doctor asked Dad what year it was, and he replied, "1949."

Then he asked, "And who is the president?"

Dad looked confident and as if he was going to answer correctly. His eyes lit up, and he began to tap the side of his head and said, "Oh, I know his name."

The doctor said, "I'll give you a hint. His first name is George."

I went through a wide range of emotions in the next few seconds. First, I was excited thinking that Dad would definitely get the answer correct now after being given that hint. Then, when he did not answer immediately, I became confused. How could he not get the answer correct now after hearing that clue? And then there was extreme fear. It suddenly occurred to me that he could very possibly answer George Washington! I held my breath while Dad searched his brain for the answer.

Finally, he replied, "I don't know who the president is."

There were more questions asked, like, "Can you repeat these three words; apple, penny, table?" Then a minute later, the doctor asked Dad to recall the three objects. He could not do it. He was asked to draw the same shapes that the doctor drew. He was not able to do it. He answered some questions correctly, but all I could focus on were the ones that seemed so easy that he got incorrect.

I could see that Dad was very embarrassed. I was devastated. His mental state was definitely worse than I thought it was. I tried to relieve his worry by telling him that my memory was not what it used to be either.

There was a brief moment of levity at the end of the test. The doctor gave Dad a piece of paper and a pen and told him to write a sentence that included a subject and a verb. It was all I could do to keep my jaw from dropping to the floor. How could this man, who did not know where he lived, how old he was, or who the president was, write a sentence. And how would he know what a subject and verb were?

Dad very proudly set to work writing his sentence. As he was scribbling away, the doctor and I looked at each other questioningly. My stomach was in knots, waiting to see the finished product.

Finally, Dad handed the paper and pen back to the doctor. When the doctor finished reading it, he began to chuckle. I could not imagine what he could be laughing at as he handed the paper to me to look at. Dad had written, "Let me out of here so I could get something to eat." Not only had he written a sentence that included a subject and verb, but he also used correct grammar, capitalizing the first letter in the sentence and putting a period at the end. I wanted to do a happy dance. I was so proud of Dad.

We waited in silence for the doctor to total his score. Out of thirty questions, Dad got twenty correct. The doctor explained that there were three levels on this test: mild, moderate, and severe. Dad scored mild but leaned toward moderate. He felt that it was still possible for him to live on his own with help.

The doctor left the examination room, and I ran after him with a list of questions that I did not want to ask in front of Dad. Was there any cure for this horrible disease? Was there another medication that Dad could try to slow the progression? What should I be looking for? What condition was he going to be in if he reached the severe stages of Alzheimer's disease? Each answer depressed me more and more. There was no cure, we could try different medications that may slow down the progression, but there was no guarantee that they would help. But the answer that stuck in my head that day and for many years after was that, should Dad live long enough to advance to the severe stages, he would most likely become incontinent and have to wear a diaper, and he may not recognize any of his loved ones.

I felt like someone reached into my chest and ripped my heart out. How could this strong, able-bodied, proud man end his life wearing a diaper? And how could this man who looked at his children like the sun rose and set on us and who loved his grandchildren with all his heart get to a point where he would not know who we were?

I remember driving home that night with tears streaming down my face. I remember praying and asking God to please take him before he got to that point. I did not want to remember my father that way. Unfortunately, that prayer was not answered.

CHAPTER 19

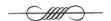

A Double-Edged Sword

One of the most difficult things to accept about Dad's Alzheimer's disease diagnosis was the fact that physically he was extremely healthy while mentally he was declining. His cholesterol level was perfect, his blood pressure was right where it should be, and he was able to walk five miles three or four times a week without batting an eye. Many times, if I was with him on those walks, I would have to plead with him to slow down as I could not keep up with him. And, like his cardiologist had told us, he was in better shape than many sixty-year-old men that he treated. I know that I should have been happy about that and thankful that he was so healthy, but it was a double-edged sword.

Because Dad was so physically healthy when he was diagnosed with Alzheimer's at eighty-five years old, there was a very good chance that he would live to advance to the severe stages of the disease. Unlike a physical illness like heart disease or cancer, in which it is clear what the cause of death is, I did not understand what causes death with Alzheimer's disease. How many years could someone live in the severe stages of this disease? I needed to find the answer to this.

I called Dad's doctor a few weeks after he had administered the MMSE and asked him to explain the stages of this disease to me further. While he had told me that Dad could very well end his life being incontinent and not recognizing anyone, what would actually cause his death? What he told me was astonishing. He said that what eventually causes someone with Alzheimer's to die was that the person no longer remembers how to swallow. I was shocked to hear this.

I thought that swallowing was a natural reflex and that it was not something that you had to "remember." After all, a baby knows how to swallow. They are not taught that. How did someone forget how to swallow? And does that mean that the person eventually starves to death? The news just kept getting worse and worse.

The doctor explained to me that as the disease progresses, it affects the area of the brain that controls swallowing. He stated that at this stage, Dad would be placed on hospice, and we would have to decide whether or not to administer a feeding tube. If we chose not to have a feeding tube inserted, Dad would be kept comfortable on morphine until his body eventually shut down due to the lack of nourishment. I was horrified to hear this news.

There is a part of me that is ashamed to write this. But if you have dealt with the degradation of Alzheimer's disease, you will understand what I am about to say. There were many times over the eight years of watching my father slip away mentally bit by bit each day that I wished he would pass away peacefully in his sleep. I loved him dearly and enjoyed any time that I had with him, but knowing what was at the end of this journey was such a painful image for me, as well as Sam. Not only did I not want to see my father be incontinent and not able to recognize the people who loved him, but the thought that he would not be able to swallow and would basically starve to death was more than I could bear. Again, I prayed that God would take him before he got to this stage.

In the fall of 2009, Dad began experiencing shortness of breath. I made an appointment with his cardiologist, and we went in to see him immediately. He examined Dad and told him that he wanted him to wear a monitor for a few days so that he could see what his heart rhythms looked like. Dad was still able to follow some directions at this time, so he knew that he had to keep the monitor on. After a few days, we went back to the cardiologist for the results.

Apparently, Dad had an irregular heartbeat. His doctor recommended a pacemaker. He said that it was a simple procedure and that he would only be in the hospital for a few days. So we made the arrangements, and Dad was admitted the following week.

The surgery went perfectly, and the pacemaker was installed. The doctor came into Dad's room the following day to explain the logistics of this new piece of equipment. He told Dad that he would have to hook up electrodes to his chest once a month and phone in to the office. They would be able to remotely monitor his heartbeat and make sure the pacemaker was doing what it was supposed to do. He also told Dad that the pacemaker battery would last for ten years.

After hearing this statement, Dad looked at the doctor and, without missing a beat, said, "Well, how do I change the battery at that point?" At the time of this surgery, Dad was eighty-nine. He obviously thought that he was still going to be here at ninety-nine to be able to change the battery in his pacemaker. The doctor and I both tried to stifle our laughter, but Dad was completely serious.

I remember thinking afterward that he could very likely live to be able to change the battery. Now that he had the pacemaker, his irregular heartbeat was taken care of. And every other aspect of his health was perfect. So maybe his question was not as far-fetched as we had thought.

Again, I was so happy that Dad was doing so well physically. But with Alzheimer's disease, it truly is a double-edged sword. While I was thankful that his physical health was so great, this meant that there would be a much better chance that he would reach that final, severe stage of this debilitating disease. I did not know what to wish for.

Dad was released from the hospital a short time after his procedure with a new lease on life. He felt great, and his heart rhythms were perfect due to the pacemaker. He was no longer experiencing shortness of breath, and he was raring to go. I remember thinking at the time that he was like the Energizer Bunny... He just kept going and going.

Sam helped Dad phone in every few weeks to check to see that the pacemaker was working well. Each time, the results were great. He was feeling terrific physically. He was back to walking five miles three or four times a week and feeling like a man half his age. But each day he was still declining mentally and sliding down the slope of Alzheimer's disease. We continued to live with the double-edged sword.

CHAPTER 20

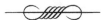

If You Don't Laugh, You'll Cry

Many of the things that Dad did as this horrible disease took over his brain left me in tears. However, some of them made me laugh and then feel guilty for laughing at him. But I think it was one of those instances in life that you have to either laugh, or you'll cry.

One of those instances happened one night when my children and I had gone out for dinner with Dad to a Chinese restaurant. Dad had poured himself a cup of tea. Before I could register what he was doing, he took the hot mustard that we had been using as a dip for our noodles and dumped it into his tea. As I was trying to form the words to stop him, he brought the cup to his lips and took a sip. I did not want to embarrass him in front of my children, who had not noticed, so I did not say anything. I assumed that he would quickly notice that his tea didn't taste very appealing. However, he continued to drink it! I refrained from saying anything because both ingredients were edible, the tea and the mustard, so I didn't think it would be harmful to him. I just would never have thought to put those two substances together.

Another laughable moment happened one day when we took my brother's dogs for a walk. Sam had two dogs at the time named Sadie and Ava. Both dogs loved my dad. As soon as they would see him, they would run up to greet him, tails wagging. And likewise, he loved them. There were numerous outings where Dad, Sam, and I went for walks, and Sadie and Ava would come along. Dad would throw the ball and have the dogs fetch it. He thoroughly enjoyed his time spent with them.

One day, we went for a walk at one of our favorite parks. Dad had been playing with the dogs and talking to them throughout the walk. At one point, he looked at me and said, "Oh, does Sam have two dogs?"

Sam and I looked at each other incredulously and had to immediately turn away because we started to laugh. Was he just realizing that there were two dogs?

I said to Sam, "Oh my god, I can't believe we're laughing at him."

Sam replied, "Yeah, but if we don't laugh, we'll cry."

He was so right.

Something that would happen on numerous occasions that would cause my whole family to laugh hysterically involved my daily routine of getting Dad to take his pills. When he was still living at home, I would fill up his pillbox once a week with his morning and evening pills. Because I was not sure that he would be able to remember to take them, I would call him every morning and evening to remind him. I would tell him what day it was and then which box to open—either morning or evening. He would have to put the phone down so that he could get a glass of water and take the pills. Easy enough, right? Except that every once in a while, he would then forget to pick the phone back up. So I would start yelling, "Dad, pick up the phone!" over and over again. I'd hear him moving around his kitchen, washing the dishes, opening and closing cabinets and drawers, talking to himself. But he could not hear me yelling to him and would never pick the phone back up.

I would wrestle with the decision to just hang up or wait until he finally realized I was on the phone. If I hung up, his phone would be off the hook, and I would not be able to contact him. But how long should I wait for him to realize he forgot about me? One time, I waited fifteen minutes, and then he just hung up the phone! This routine happened at least once a week. It made for some hearty laughter in my household.

During the course of Dad's decline, I took on the job of doing his grocery shopping. I realized I needed to do this when I opened his cupboard one day and found eight boxes of Corn Flakes. Each time he went grocery shopping, he brought home another box. On one of my shopping excursions, I noticed that the treats that Sam gave to Sadie and Ava were on sale, so I decided to buy a box of them. I wasn't going to see Sam for a while, so I left the box at Dad's with the instructions for him to give them to Sam when he came to visit that week.

Sam called me a few days later, trying hard to speak through his laughter. He had just had a phone conversation with Dad in which he was raving about the new "snacks" that I had purchased for him. When Sam asked him what they were, Dad told him he wasn't sure, but the box said, "Snausages". Horrified, Sam asked what was on the box, and Dad told him that there was a dog on the front. Sam immediately told him to throw the box in the trash.

On another shopping trip, I had purchased bananas for Dad, which he loved. I was not going to be able to make another trip to his house that week, so I decided to stock him up until I could get there again the following week. I bought thirteen bananas. Some were yellow and some were a little green. I thought that over the course of the week, the green ones would ripen, and he'd be well stocked.

Sam went to visit Dad the next day. When he got there, he called and asked me if I needed him to do anything for Dad while he was there. I told him that I had done his wash, cleaned, and grocery shopped, so there was nothing that he needed to do. Sam then asked me why I had not gotten any bananas when I grocery shopped.

"What do you mean?" I asked. "I bought thirteen of them yesterday when I went to the grocery store."

"Well, there are none here now," Sam said. A feeling of dread crept over me.

"Sam," I said. "Check the trash can."

Sam looked in the trash can and found thirteen banana peels. Dad had eaten all the bananas in one day!

I felt sick. I knew that bananas had potassium, but I did not know if too much potassium was harmful. So I quickly did some research. I found that too much of it can lead to an irregular heartbeat, stomach pain, and diarrhea. But even more concerning than that was that too much potassium could lead to a sometimes-fatal condition called hyperkalemia.

I immediately got on the phone to call Dad's doctor. When he called me back, he reassured me that he would had to have eaten many more than thirteen bananas in a day for it to have any serious implications. But he did tell us to keep an eye on him for the stomach pain and diarrhea that he may get. Sam stayed with Dad that night to make sure that he was alright. Luckily, he was fine. But I would no longer be buying that many bananas on our shopping trips.

The same thing happened when I decided to buy Dad his favorite candy, a Hershey chocolate bar with almonds. I had been in a store and seen a giant-sized bar that was seven ounces. I thought this would be good for Dad because he could break off little pieces, and it would last him a while. Wrong. I purchased it for him and left it at his house. When I called him the next morning, he said, "Baby doll, thank you for that Hershey bar. It was so good."

Dread crept through me at the word "was."

I said, "Dad, how much of the candy bar did you eat?"

He casually replied, "The whole thing."

Not wanting to draw attention to the fact that he had eaten 1,089 calories, seventy-one grams of fat, and eighty-seven grams of sugar in one sitting, I casually asked him how he felt.

"I feel great," he said.

I was in shock. How could he have eaten all that chocolate and sugar and not be feeling sick. I immediately got off the phone and called the doctor again. He assured me that he would be okay, but he may feel a little sick and would, most likely, not be able to sleep that night after consuming all that sugar. When I called the next morning and asked Dad how he felt and if he had slept, he told me that he felt great and that he had slept like a baby. I was so relieved. But like the bananas, I would not be buying large candy bars any longer.

As Dad continued to decline, so did his ability to have meaningful conversations. He could answer simple questions, and he could definitely ask questions, sometimes asking the same question ten times in the course of an hour. However, he could not hold up his end of an in-depth conversation.

The lack of this ability became very apparent whenever we would go somewhere in the car. Where, before his Alzheimer's disease progression, he had been able to converse about the news, the weather, or the kids, now there was just silence—well, until he discovered road signs, that is.

Instead of sitting in silence during our many car rides, Dad began reading all the signs along the side of the road. So his "conversations" went like this: "Right lane must turn right." "Forty-five miles per hour." "Yield." When this first started, I was not sure if I should comment or just let Dad read and stay silent. Then he began adding commentary after reading some of the signs, and I had to refrain from laughing. He would say, "Forty-five miles per hour, what the hell?" or "No right turn, why not?"

I'm ashamed to admit that I found myself driving faster so that Dad would not be able to read all the signs along our route. But the only thing that did was cause him to read faster. Sometimes I would start up a conversation to try to divert Dad's attention away from the signs. But he would just continue to read them while I was speaking.

I finally learned to accept that this was another phase of his disease that he could not control. Long car rides were very difficult and would sometimes result in my turning on the radio to drown out all the "Forty-five miles per hour, what the hells" along our route. I eventually got to the point that I could just tune it out. Earplugs helped!

Some of Dad's conversations with us were so strange that we had no idea how to reply. One day, after he had gone on one of his long walks, he called me to tell me what had happened. Apparently, according to him, there was an airplane that was following him as he was walking. He felt that someone had given the pilot instructions to follow him, and Dad felt that the orders came "from the president on down." He was adamant that this had happened, and he felt threatened and could not understand why he was being followed.

I tried to reassure him that there was no one following him and that it was probably just a coincidence that the airplane was flying over him, but there was no altering his thinking. After several attempts to put his mind to rest, I just decided to change the subject and move on to talking about the weather. Then I called Sam to discuss Dad's latest comical discussion. We laughed at the absurdity of him thinking that the president had ordered a pilot to follow him. But inside, I wanted to cry over the fact that he actually thought this. And that he was actually feeling fear. It was the usual battle of emotions that I felt.

Through all these changes in Dad's behavior that we found ourselves laughing at, the emotion that would immediately follow would be guilt—guilt at laughing at Dad for carrying out these strange behaviors that left us scratching our heads. However, we soon came to realize that the saying, "If you don't laugh, you'll cry" is such an apt quote for what we were experiencing. While it was hard seeing our father acting in these peculiar ways, the laughter helped us to get through it and keep going along this path with him. And we also realized that had Dad been his old normal self with the wonderful sense of humor that he had, he would have had a good laugh at some of his own odd behaviors. This helped to alleviate the guilt we were feeling.

CHAPTER 21

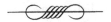

Correcting Him

One of the hardest things I could not seem to get through my head about Dad's Alzheimer's disease was the fact that I should just go along with whatever he said. There were so many times that he said things that just shocked me. So instead of nodding and going along with it, I would correct him. This led to frustration, embarrassment, and sadness on Dad's part and guilt on mine.

One such occasion happened the morning my father called to tell me of his plans for the day. He was going to get in the car and drive to New Jersey to visit his brother Joe. The problem with this was that my uncle Joe had died fifteen years prior to that.

I listened in astonishment as my dad said that he was going to go visit his brother for the day, and he would be back later that evening.

I said, "Dad, Uncle Joe died."

And my father's response ripped my heart out. "He died? What do you mean he died?" he mournfully exclaimed.

I gently replied, "Dad, he died a while ago."

With his voice cracking, he said, "I didn't know he died. And I didn't even go to his funeral."

I tried to reassure him that he was with Uncle Joe at the end and that he was at his funeral, but he just broke down. It was a horrible phone call that left me feeling like a wretched person who had given my dad shocking news. And obviously news that, in his confused mind, he was hearing for the first time.

I remember a friend telling me the story of his grandmother who had Alzheimer's disease and would search for her deceased husband every night, only to be told by her family each night that her husband had died. He stated that it was as if she lost him all over again each time they relayed this news to her. It was not until much later that they realized that they should have just said that he was away and that he would be back soon. This would have saved her much anguish.

I should have done the same thing with my dad the day he said he was going to visit Uncle Joe. I could have just said that Uncle Joe was away and that he should postpone his trip to another day when he would be home. Dad would have forgotten about it until the next time he got this idea, and I would have to divert him again. Instead, my news brought him heartache.

Dad was losing all concept of time and place at this point, so there were many times that he would state something incorrectly, and I found myself correcting him. There were many occasions when he would say it was a beautiful morning, and it would clearly be evening. He would call me at 7:00 p.m. and say that he had just gotten up, thinking that it was 7:00 a.m. I would correct him and tell him that it was 7:00 p.m., and he would respond with a chuckle and say, "Oh yeah, that's right."

The seasons were another area where I found myself correcting Dad. We would head out for one of our long walks breathing in the crisp autumn air with leaves crunching under our feet when Dad would proclaim, "I just love the springtime."

Of course, I would have to say, "Dad, it's autumn. Do you see the leaves on the ground?"

To which he would reply, "Oh yeah, that's right."

I could see the embarrassment on his face, which would then make me feel awful.

One of the many facets of Alzheimer's disease is the repetition of statements and stories. Someone with the disease could repeat the same sentence over and over in a short interval of time. This happened on many occasions with Dad. We could be sitting and having a conversation, and he would repeat the same statement, verbatim, five to ten times. Often, I found myself saying, "I know, Dad, you already told me that."

And he would reply, "Oh, right, I already said that."

But I'm not sure he really remembered saying it previously.

My husband told me repeatedly to just go along with whatever Dad said. I would get so mad at myself when I saw the embarrassment on his face when I corrected him. I would berate myself and swear that I was not going to do it the next time. But after doing some soul searching to try to figure out why I continued to do it, I finally came to the realization that I was desperately just trying to bring my dad back to reality. I think I thought that by correcting him, I could snap him out of it, and we could have the conversations that we used to have, where he made sense and he did not repeat himself, and he knew time and place and knew that his brother had died. And when he did not have Alzheimer's disease.

CHAPTER 22

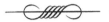

Here We Go Again

As I stated, one of the many facets of Alzheimer's disease is the constant repetition. This could include repeating the same story over and over, asking the same question within minutes of receiving the answer, or the ceaseless stating of a phrase. The first few times it happens it can be somewhat annoying. However, when you spend a significant amount of time with a person who does this, you will do anything to get them to stop the repetitive remarks. I found myself doing this frequently with Dad.

On our many walks at the various parks that we would visit, a common phrase that Dad would repeat over and over was, "It's so nice to get a whiff of this fresh air." It was wonderful to hear him say that and to see the enjoyment on his face as we were hiking. For the first ten times that he said it, that is. However, after that, I would find myself grinding my teeth and finding ways to steer the conversation to something other than the fresh air.

Another common phrase was, "It feels so good to get this sun on my face." Again, I was very happy to see Dad enjoying the simple things in life like the sun and fresh air. But the phrase became irritating after hearing it about twenty times during the course of our walk. I felt that maybe it was because he did not have much going on in his life at this point, and he was trying to make conversation. So we would talk about Jimmy and Katelyn, what they were doing in school, how Jim was doing, how Sam's job was going, and countless other subjects. But in the end, he would again declare, "It's so nice to get a whiff of this fresh air."

I would reply, "It sure is, Dad," for the umpteenth time.

Dad's hearing had gotten progressively worse over the years. Sam and I found ourselves having to yell so that he was able to hear us speak to him. This became embarrassing in restaurants as people thought we were raising our voices to him in anger. Dad swore that his hearing problems were due to the war and the constant sounds of gunfire and bombs going off. So I contacted the Veterans Administration and asked if they could offer him any help. They stated that, because he was a veteran, he was entitled to receive free hearing aids. Dad had tried them previously and found that they did not work. However, the Veterans Administration was offering the most advanced hearing aids on the market made with the latest technology. We made an appointment for Dad at the Veterans Administration Audiology Department.

I explained this to Dad and told him that he was getting these hearing aids because he was a veteran. I assured him that they would help him to hear better. He was very receptive to this as he knew that he was missing out on so much due to his hearing loss. So we embarked on our trip to the Veterans Administration to get him fitted for his new hearing aids.

When we got there, they took a mold of Dad's ears and informed us that they would be custom made to fit him perfectly. They would be ready in about two weeks. And the best part was that this was not going to cost Dad a thing, which made him very happy.

Two weeks later, we went back to the Veterans Administration hospital, and Dad was fitted with his new hearing aids. As soon as they were placed in his ears, I very quietly said, "Dad, can you hear me?"

And he replied, "Yes, I can hear you."

I got tears of happiness in my eyes as I realized that we would no longer have to raise our voices in order for Dad to hear us. We left the VA with the new hearing aids in his ears and a year's supply of batteries for them. I was so excited as we got in the car to drive home.

As we began our journey home, I talked to Dad in a normal tone of voice, and he could hear every word I said. We talked about how thrilled we were that the hearing aids seemed to be helping him. We also talked about how wonderful it was that he was able to take advantage of this amazing benefit for veterans. We were both smiling about his newfound ability to hear.

Ten minutes into our ride, Dad turned to me and asked, "What are these plugs in my ears?"

I looked over at him in astonishment. "Dad, they are the hearing aids that we just discussed. They are going to help you hear, and you didn't have to pay anything for them because of the fact that you are a veteran. Remember I told you about this?"

He looked at me and said, "Oh, that's right. You did tell me about that. Now I remember."

I drew a sigh of relief.

Ten minutes later, we were discussing another topic when Dad looked at me once again and said, "What are these plugs in my ears?"

I was not sure whether to laugh or cry. I tried to remain patient as I again answered, "Dad, they are the new hearing aids that you were given by the Veterans Administration. Remember how we talked about how your hearing has deteriorated and how, because you are a veteran, you are entitled to free hearing aids to help you with your hearing loss?"

"Oh, that's right," he said.

I was cautiously optimistic that I had finally gotten through to him. That is, until he once again asked me about the plugs in his ears a half hour later. I gave up trying to explain it.

Unfortunately, the hearing aids did not last very long. Dad never understood what the "plugs" were and constantly took them out of his ears. We found them in his pockets, stuffed in a drawer, and in countless other places. So rather than have to continually explain it to him and constantly having to look for them, we just put them away and went back to speaking very loudly to him.

These types of repetitive conversations happened regularly over the course of Dad's disease. They required massive amounts of patience on the part of Sam and I as we tried to converse with Dad. One such conversation happened every time that Dad and I would go to his favorite park for our walks.

There were certain landmarks along the way from Dad's house to the park that he acknowledged with the same comments each and every time that we made the drive. The comments went like this:

As we came to the traffic light, leaving Dad's neighborhood, he would look to his right and say, "Boy, you know, that telephone pole is really leaning. They should fix that."

After we made the turn and were driving down the road for a little while, Dad would look to his right and comment about how crowded the apartment complex was. The first ten times or so, I corrected him and told him that it was not an apartment complex but an office complex. Then I realized that it was pointless to correct him, so I let it go.

Next came a used car lot. Each time we would come to this lot, the script went like this, "Boy, you know, sometimes when you go by this lot, there are a ton of cars there, and sometimes when you go by, there's not a one."

Never in all the years that I had driven by this car lot had I ever seen it empty. But, obviously, Dad thought that he had seen that, so I just went along with it. What was the use in arguing?

Next on our trip was the bank on the corner. It had many glass windows, which Dad thought was terrible construction for a bank, and he made this known each time we passed it. The next landmark that Dad would comment on was the hospital that was being built.

"You know, I just read in the newspaper this morning that they are building a hospital over there."

The hospital took two years to build, but each time we drove by, he said that he had just read in the newspaper that morning that they were building a hospital in that location.

Finally, as we were turning into the park, Dad would comment on the new office building that was built on the corner.

"You know, they just moved that building here. There was nothing on that spot for the longest time, and now they moved that building and placed it on that lot."

The building was built there, not moved there, but, again, what was the use in disagreeing with him?

By this point in our trip, I had nodded, smiled, and agreed with him at least five times. And I could have recited the script verbatim as it never varied. Dad said the exact same thing each time we made this journey. It was as if a recording was being played every time we set out on this route.

One day, I decided to discuss it with Sam. I asked, "When you leave Dad's neighborhood with him, does he say anything as you're traveling along the route?"

I sat in silent awe as Sam recited, word for word, the exact narration that I encountered each time. By the time Sam got to the hospital being built, we both recited, in unison, "You know, I just read in the newspaper this morning that they are building a hospital there."

Again, we laughed as we realized he said the exact same thing to both of us each time he made that trip.

I decided to check with Barbara to see if she noticed the same thing. And, to my amazement, he said the same things to her when they set out on their journeys together. I decided to do some research to try to figure out if this was a common symptom of Alzheimer's disease.

According to Ira Hyman, PhD, a professor of psychology at Western Washington University, this repetitive phrasing is called a conversation loop, and it is typical of a person with Alzheimer's disease. The patient gets stuck in this loop because they do not remember that they have had the conversation. They get stuck on repeat, repeating the topic multiple times during the course of a conversation. Maybe even returning to the topic over several days, or as in our case, over multiple days.

I learned that when this repetitive behavior occurred, the best thing to do was to redirect the person. Because they get stuck in this loop, by redirecting them to another topic, it may help them to get out of the "loop" and focus on another topic. I followed a blog in which people experiencing the same repetitive conversations suggested ways to handle it. One person stated that they interrupt the loop by stepping in several seconds ahead of what the Alzheimer's patient is thinking. Another blogger suggested bringing up the past, which is sometimes easier for the patient to remember than the present.

I tried this new approach with Dad, and it helped. When he would ask me the same question that I had just answered five minutes ago, instead of answering him, I would ask him to tell me about when he lived in Philadelphia with his family. He would start to talk about it, and the conversation would be steered in another direction. This helped me immensely with my patience in dealing with Dad.

I also found myself starting a conversation about something from his past before we got to the landmarks on our journey. As we approached the first landmark, I would say, "Dad, tell me about your life on the farm. What was a typical day like on the Valenti farm?"

By starting this dialogue, his mind was steered in another direction, and he would not begin the loop that he recited each time we drove that route. I would try to direct his attention to something besides the telephone pole, the office complex, the used car lot, the bank, the hospital being built, etc. Anything so that I would not have to hear the repetitive loop again and risk losing my patience. It was an exercise in survival on my part.

CHAPTER 23

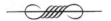

Carol

The game plan that Sam and I had put into place for Dad's care seemed to be working out fine. We each visited twice a week and took care of his grocery shopping, cleaning, wash, bill paying, yard work, doctor's visits, and errands. Barbara came three afternoons a week and took him out for walks and provided companionship. However, there were still voids in his day that we wanted to fill. So, once again, we set out to find help.

I contacted the agency that found Barbara for us. I told them that we were looking for someone to cover a few hours two days a week. We wanted someone on the days that Barbara was not there to just provide companion care for Dad. They recommended a woman named Carol.

Sam and I met with Carol the following week and were both impressed with the energetic, lively, elderly woman that we met with. We explained exactly what we were looking for with regards to care for Dad. We told her that we wanted her to come on Tuesday and Thursday for about three hours to take him out to get something to eat or for a walk. She seemed very amendable to our requirements and said that she could start the following week. We were so happy to know that we had found another person to help with Dad's care.

Carol visited Dad every Tuesday and Thursday from 12:00 p.m. to 3:00 p.m. She took him for walks or to the nearby mall, which he loved. He also loved just going to grocery stores and walking around, looking at everything. Just like Barbara, she left a detailed written message for me every time she was there highlighting what they had done that day. Dad seemed to be thoroughly enjoying his time with Carol. We felt so lucky to have two such wonderful women taking care of our father when we could not be there.

As time went on, Carol suggested taking Dad to the local senior center. We thought that this was a wonderful idea. He could socialize with people his age, and it would be another activity to get him out of the house. So every Tuesday and Thursday, Dad and Carol would head out to the senior center where Dad would play cards with some of the men, and they would have lunch together. They also had an exercise class there called Silver Sneakers that Dad enjoyed participating in. He took part in all the seasonal activities held there, such as the Halloween parade, in which Dad dressed up as the Tin Man from the *Wizard of Oz*, thanks to Carol's creativity. There were also many field trips that the senior center went on for the day. Carol would accompany Dad on these adventures to the casinos in Atlantic City, local farms, and community fairs. They both seemed to be enjoying this time together.

Over the years that Carol was with Dad, we started to notice her slipping a little bit. She would forget things I asked her to do, show up late, or show up on a day that she was not supposed to. This happened one particular day, and it caused a tremendous amount of angst.

Barbara had arrived at Dad's house at her regular time on Wednesday and knocked on his door. There was no answer. She kept knocking, and when he did not answer after several attempts, she began looking in the windows. She saw a pair of his sneakers by the sofa, which caused her alarm because she felt that if his sneakers were there, he must be at home. She tried calling his phone, but there was no answer. She began to get scared.

Barbara called me at work to tell me what was going on. I tried calling Sam to see if he knew where Dad could be, but he didn't know. I told Barbara to go around to the backyard and see if he was, perhaps, doing some gardening. He wasn't. By this time, an hour had gone by, and we had no idea where he was. Terrible thoughts started going through my mind. Did he fall in another room, and Barbara could not see him through the window? Was he passed out somewhere in the house? I decided to call my brother-in-law who was a policeman in Dad's township.

When I explained to him what was going on, he went over to investigate. He walked all around the house, looking in the windows and calling out Dad's name. After searching and not having any luck, he called me and asked if he should break into the house. I told him to break down the door.

Just as he was getting ready to do that, Carol pulled into the driveway with Dad in the passenger's seat. My brother-in-law handed his phone to Carol, and I asked her what was going on. She very calmly explained that she had taken Dad out for a walk.

"Carol, it's not your day to visit with Dad," I said.

And she replied, "Yes, it is. It's Tuesday."

After some explaining from myself and Barbara, she finally realized that it was Wednesday and not her day to be there. She seemed very confused and upset. I assured her that it was an honest mistake, but this mistake had caused us a great deal of fear.

There were a few more of these incidents as time went on, and then I finally realized that Carol may be experiencing Alzheimer's disease herself. I did not feel that it was safe to have her still caring for Dad, so I explained to her that we were going to make other arrangements for him. She was not pleased about this, but I had to do what was right and safe for my father. It was time to look for someone else to take Carol's place. Along came another angel sent from above.

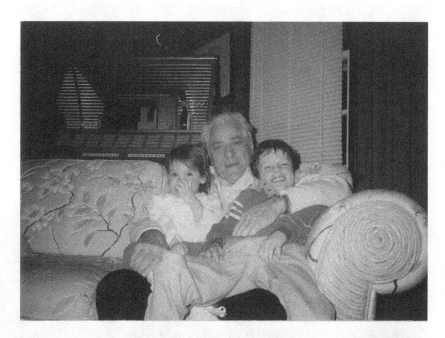

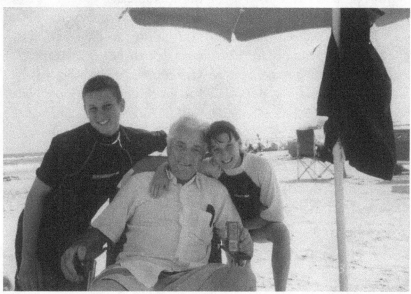

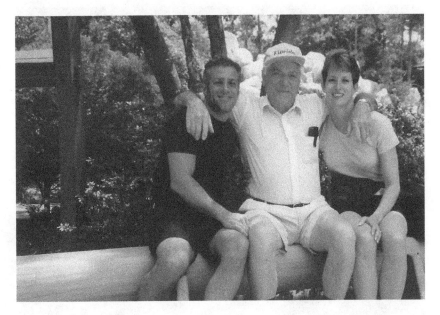

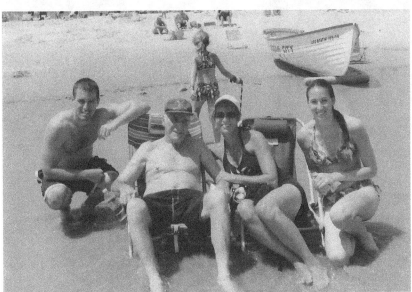

Dad was always happy to spend time with his family

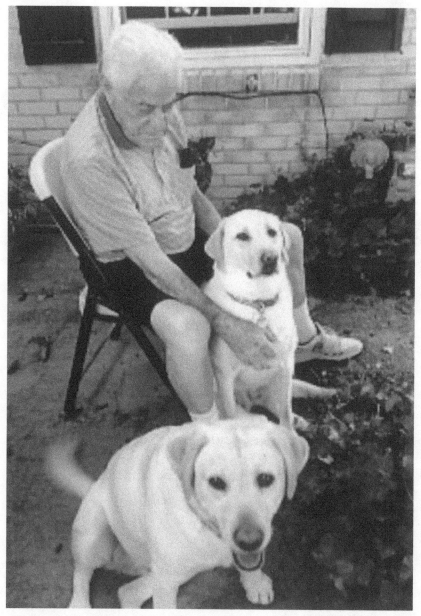

Dad with Sadie and Ava

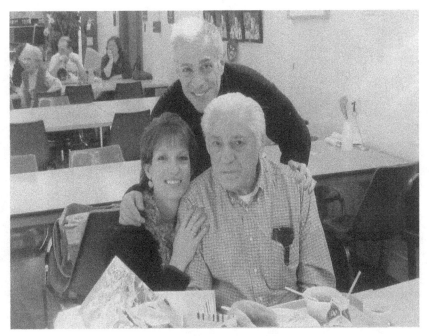

Celebrating Dad's 90th birthday at the Senior Center.
The look of confusion on his face was starting to replace
his beautiful smile at this stage of the disease.

CHAPTER 24

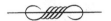

Carla

Once again, Sam and I set out to find a nurturing, caring, kind person to help us take care of Dad. We posted an advertisement on a site specifically for caregivers, and we received many responses. We looked through their credentials and picked about five or six people to interview. We set up the interviews over a two-day period. Sam and I came up with a list of questions and requirements for our interviewees, and we met each of them at a coffee shop and began our interviewing process.

Halfway through the second day, we were starting to lose hope. None of the candidates were a good fit for Dad and the schedule that we had come up with. We had one more person to interview before we were going to head back to the drawing board.

As we sat waiting in the coffee shop, Sam and I were feeling a little discouraged. This was not going the way we had hoped. And then in walked a breath of fresh air. A woman came strolling through the door with a wave and a huge smile that lit up the coffee shop. She came up to Sam and me, gave each of us a hug, and told us that her name was Carla. We could not wait to interview this charismatic woman.

We went through our list of questions, and she answered every one perfectly. We asked her why she thought she would be a good caregiver for our father. Her answer brought me to tears. She told us that she had lost her elderly father, whom she had cared for for many years, the year before, and she missed him very much. When she had seen our ad for a caregiver for an elderly man, she felt like it was God's work putting us together. We were sold.

We went over the schedule that we wanted her to work, and she was agreeable to exactly what we needed for Dad. She asked us if we would be okay with her taking him to any local fairs, parades, or festivals that were being held, and we agreed wholeheartedly. Many times, when Sam and I were visiting Dad, we were so busy taking care of his lawn, the bills, cleaning, grocery shopping, and general housekeeping chores that we were not able to do "fun" things with him. So we were thrilled that Carla was proposing these fun activities to entertain him.

She started right away. She was with Dad on Tuesday and Thursday afternoons, and Barbara continued her Monday, Wednesday, and Friday schedule. On many occasions, Carla brought along her young grandson on the excursions that she and Dad went on. Dad had always loved interacting with children, so this was a welcome addition for him. He would tell us about his fun days with Carla and her grandson, Christopher, and he would always have a funny story to relay.

As Carla spent more and more time with Dad, she grew to love him and began calling him her "Sammy Sam." She would give him a big hug and kiss, and he would beam when he saw her. On one occasion, Carla had stopped by her house with Dad to pick something up, and he met Carla's mother and her neighbors. After a lively conversation with all of them, they asked Carla to start bringing him by more often to visit. She began doing this on a regular basis, and he thoroughly enjoyed the socializing that this afforded him. Likewise, Carla's mom and friends grew to love Dad and looked forward to these outings.

Carla would often look up the calendar of community activities. She would find parades, picnics, festivals, ice-cream socials, and many other fun things for she and Dad to do. Many times, he would relay to me what he and Carla did that day and how much he enjoyed it. But as his disease progressed, I would ask him if he had fun with Carla that day, only to get the response, "Carla? No, Carla wasn't here today?" I would be looking at the picture that Carla had texted me of the two of them eating ice-cream cones that day at a community picnic as Dad was telling me he had not seen Carla in a while. At least he seemed to be having a great time at the moment the picture was taken, even if he could not remember it later.

Along with taking him to many events, Carla would sit outside on Dad's patio with him and read the newspaper and play cards. He had always loved playing cards, and even when his memory failed him in other areas, he seemed to remember the card game "War" whenever they played. Dad also loved caring for a garden, so Carla helped him to plant tomatoes in the spring and then tend to the garden throughout the summer. As his disease progressed, he no longer had an interest in gardening and could not seem to follow the rules of the card game anymore.

Carla was with Dad for three years and had seen him decline sharply during that time. She often said that she wished she had known him before he had Alzheimer's disease because she would have loved to have had deeper conversations with him and gotten to know him better. As it was, what she had gotten to know about him, she grew to love very much. And he, in turn, loved her. She had expressed to me on many occasions that whenever she was feeling down, she would pick Dad up for one of their excursions, and her Sammy Sam would lift her spirits with his huge smile and his usual comment, "What a beautiful day to get out for some fresh air and a walk." She was amazed at how every day was a positive day for him and how much he enjoyed the simple things in life, like being outside, the sunshine, and the fresh air.

Carla told us on many occasions that Dad would always have a special place in her heart. I know she held a special place in his, as well as Sam's and mine. We felt so blessed and fortunate to have added this wonderful woman to our caregiving team.

CHAPTER 25

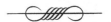

Driver's License

Over the course of Dad's decline, there were many things that we had to take away from him. I took over paying his bills since he could no longer keep track of which ones he had paid, Sam took over cutting his grass, and when he could get there after a snowstorm, Sam took care of the snow shoveling. The grocery shopping, cleaning, doctor's appointments, laundry, preparing meals; all these activities of daily living were things that we had to take away from him as his Alzheimer's disease got worse. We felt that he could no longer do them sufficiently or safely. However, perhaps one of the hardest things we had to do during the course of Dad's disease was to take away his driver's license.

When he was about eighty-eight, I had gotten a disturbing phone call from a police officer telling me that Dad had not stopped for a school bus in the opposite lane that was picking up children. He told me that we might want to consider talking to his doctor about pulling his license. The officer was going to send the report to the Department of Motor Vehicles, and most likely, Dad would have to retake his driver's test.

I called Dad's doctor the next day to discuss it with him. He stated that Dad would probably not be able to pass the driver's test at this point, so to go ahead and let him take it. If he did not pass, I would not be the bad guy who was taking his license away. I thought this was a great idea. We waited for the notice to come from the

Department of Motor Vehicles requiring him to retake his driver's test.

When it came, I explained to Dad that he would have to study for the driver's test and take both the written and driving part of the test. He was very upset. He felt that he could pass the driving part without a problem. However, he was concerned about passing the written part. He understood that if he did not pass, he would have to relinquish his license, which greatly upset him. We went to the local DMV to pick up a Driver's Manual, and Dad began to study.

I was torn. I secretly prayed that he would not pass the test so that we could take his license, and he would not be a threat to himself or others on the road. But I knew that this was going to be so difficult for Dad to accept. This was yet another form of independence that would be taken away from him. This would also mean that he would be housebound until one of us could get there to take him out. I did not know what to pray for.

Dad studied hard for the test for many weeks. When the big day finally came, Sam took him to the DMV and waited in the waiting room with the other "expectant parents." He called me and told me that Dad was going to have to take the "written" part on a computer, which there was most likely no way that he would be able to navigate. He also talked about the irony of the situation. Dad had taken Sam for his driver's test twenty-seven years before at this same DMV. It was truly the circle of life.

An hour later, Sam called me with the news. Dad had passed his test with flying colors. I was so proud of him. But I was also afraid of him being on the road. It became apparent that he was a hazard on the road when he drove with Jim one day and proceeded to go through a red light without even looking. How was I going to take his license away when he had just passed the test?

We sat down with Dad and discussed the fact that he was getting older, and his memory and reflexes were not what they used to be. We told him that while he was still technically able to drive since he had passed his test, we thought that it would be better if he just waited for Sam, Barbara, Carla, or myself to take him where he needed to go. I think that his pride would not allow him to admit that he should not drive any longer. But, in the end, he drove less and less as time went on. He waited for us to take him to the places he wanted to go. And between the team that we had put in place, there were enough of us getting him out of the house so that he was not housebound. This arrangement worked well until Dad was almost ninety.

After a doctor appointment, in which Dad could not answer many of the questions that the physician asked him, he told us that he was going to recommend to the Department of Motor Vehicles that Dad's license be relinquished. There was a mixture of relief and dread as I looked at Dad and saw his face fall. His final piece of independence was being taken away from him, and it broke my heart.

We didn't discuss it after we left the appointment because I did not want to upset him any more than he was. And in a few days, he forgot about it anyway. That is the beauty of Alzheimer's disease. You forget the bad things too.

When the papers arrived from the DMV, stating that Dad had a month to send in his license, I felt sick to my stomach. It was December, and he had to send it back before the 31st. For some reason, Sam and I decided to tell Dad on Christmas Day. I do not recall why other than maybe we thought having his whole family around to support him would be a good thing. However, it was an awful Christmas memory.

I still remember sitting at the kitchen table and telling him the news. He looked so beaten and forlorn. He said, "I fought for freedom in this country, and now my freedom is being taken away." I felt like someone had stabbed me in the heart. I reassured him that he would not be housebound, that between all of us, he would still be out all the time. He said he was going to feel like a burden, and we reassured him that he was not and that we were happy to drive him wherever he needed to go.

As he opened his wallet and pulled his driver's license out to give it to me, he looked like he was going to cry. And when he handed it to me, I felt like the most horrible person in the world. This independent, strong man who had spent countless hours teaching me how to drive and parallel park to perfection, who cheered me on as I took my driving test, who had been driving since he was sixteen years old and had driven for nearly seventy-four years was handing me his last bit of independence. Life just was not fair.

As I said, the beauty of Alzheimer's disease is that the sufferer forgets the bad as well as the good. Dad did not remember the next day that we had taken his license. In order to take his car away so he would not continue to drive it, we explained to him that Sam needed to borrow it for a while since his own car was not working. Ever the helpful father that he was, he gladly gave Sam the keys and told him to keep it as long as he needed it.

Another feature of Alzheimer's disease that can be a blessing in certain situations is losing track of time. Sam told Dad that his car was still in the shop, and he needed to borrow his car a little longer, and Dad was fine with that. He had no idea that it had been three weeks since we took the car. He was not missing driving, and he was getting out just as much as he had previously, so he wasn't even asking for the car. In time, we just stopped talking about it, and Dad forgot about it. However, I never forgot the horrendous feeling of taking that piece of my father's independence from him. It was one of the worst days of my life.

CHAPTER 26

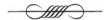

Dad's Stroke

Thanksgiving of 2010 started out like all of our Thanksgivings. I got up that morning and put our fifteen-pound turkey in the oven. Then I began getting everything else ready for our Thanksgiving dinner with Sam and Dad.

Sam was going to pick Dad up around 3:00 p.m. and come to our house for dinner at 5:00 p.m. My phone rang at 3:05 p.m.

Sam said, "Something isn't right with Dad."

"What do you mean?" I asked.

Sam went on to describe to me what was going on.

Apparently, Dad's right arm and leg were shaking uncontrollably. I asked Sam if he thought we should take him to the hospital. He was not exactly sure what was going on, so he said he would bring him to my house, and then we could decide.

When they got there, I immediately saw what Sam was talking about. Dad's right arm and leg were shaking, and he could not seem to control them. I asked him if he was okay, and he said he felt fine. I told him that I thought we should go to the hospital. He became very agitated and said that he felt fine and did not want to go to the hospital.

I called Dad's doctor and described what was happening. He said that it did not sound like anything serious but to keep an eye on it throughout the day. I asked him if it could be a stroke, and he said that if he had experienced a stroke, he would have paralysis. He said that a stroke did not usually manifest itself in the symptoms that I was describing. The doctor did not seem concerned, so we decided to go on with our day.

During dinner, I noticed Dad tucking his right leg behind the chair leg to try to stop the movement. His arm was not shaking as much as it had been earlier, so he was able to feed himself. I kept watching him and asking him if he was okay which, I could tell, was making him upset. So I stopped asking.

When it came time for Sam and Dad to leave, the tremors had seemed to subside a bit. However, Sam told me that he was going to stay with Dad that night to keep an eye on him. I felt much better, knowing Dad would not be alone.

The next morning, the shaking had gotten worse. Sam and I decided that Dad needed to go to the hospital whether he liked it or not. So I went to his house to explain that we needed to go get his shaking evaluated. He was not pleased, but he agreed to go.

We went to the emergency room and waited for two hours before a doctor saw him. The doctor seemed confused about what was happening with Dad. Like Dad's general practitioner, whom I had spoken to the previous day, he did not feel that it was a stroke. However, he could not diagnose exactly what was taking place. So the doctor decided to put him on a drug to stop the shaking and calm him down.

We had always noticed that Dad had a strange tolerance to medication. It seemed like whenever he took medication for something, the symptoms worsened instead of getting better. That's exactly what happened that day in the emergency room.

A little while after Dad was administered the drug, he began writhing uncontrollably on the gurney that he was lying on. Now not only were his right arm and leg shaking, but his whole body was also. I tried to talk to him soothingly to get him to calm down, but to no avail. He was thrashing wildly and yelling and groaning.

I told the nurses to get the doctor immediately because, obviously, he was having an adverse reaction. When the doctor came into the room and observed what was happening, he said he had never seen that reaction before. Apparently, the medication he was given belongs to the benzodiazepines class that is used to relieve anxiety and cause drowsiness. Obviously, it was not doing that for Dad.

The doctor decided to try increasing the dosage. I looked at him incredulously.

"Are you sure that's a good idea?" I asked him.

In my opinion, the reaction he was having meant that this was not the proper medicine for him. But what did I know? I had no medical experience and trusted that the doctor was correct.

More of the drug was administered to Dad. A short time later, he looked like a man possessed. He was writhing and thrashing even more than before, and now he would not stay on the bed. We tried to hold him down and calm him, but his agitation had increased tenfold.

At this point, nurses and doctors were coming in to try to calm him down. I went into the hall and called his family doctor to explain what was going on. He agreed that Dad was having an adverse reaction to the drug. He was going to confer with the emergency room doctor and see if they could come up with a different plan for his care.

After the doctors' conversation, the emergency room doctor came into the room and told us that they were going to try another drug therapy, but that they were going to admit Dad so that they could observe him overnight. The doctor felt that at his age (he was ninety at the time) the shaking and agitation were detrimental to his heart.

A little while after they admitted him, they administered the new medication. We waited with bated breath in the hopes that Dad would finally stop thrashing. At this point, it had been well over twenty-four hours that he had been doing this. How much longer could his body and heart endure this? We were about to find out.

Visiting hours at the hospital were now over, and we were told that we had to leave. I was not about to leave Dad alone in this condition. So I requested a personal aide to stay with him through the night. I had learned that this service was available to at-risk patients on another occasion that Dad was in the hospital. Hospitals will not offer the service, so the family has to insist on it or in many cases, fight for it. That is what I did that evening.

We waited until the aide arrived and left with the assurance from the doctor that this new drug was very affective on most people, and Dad should be calming down very soon. I prayed that he was right.

When I arrived at the hospital the next morning, I was appalled. Dad was being restrained by two nurses while the doctor was giving him an injection. Again, he was thrashing wildly and moaning. The aide that was with him overnight looked like she had been through a battle. With tears streaming down my face, I pulled the doctor into the hallway and asked him what was happening.

Dad had not slept all night and had continued to shake and thrash. The medication that was effective on "most" people had not worked. Apparently, Dad was not "most" people. This doctor, like the emergency room doctor from the previous day, had never seen anything like this. He said that the two injections that Dad had been given should have knocked him out. This also seemed to be having an adverse effect on him. Instead of calming him down, it was making him extremely agitated.

I felt helpless and at a loss as to what to do for Dad. I spent that whole day speaking to doctors, nurses, anyone that could give me advice on what to do to help him. The doctors tried other medications that they thought would help. I tried talking soothingly to Dad and rubbing his head and face to calm him. He would calm down for a little while and then get agitated again. During this time, he was still thrashing and having tremors.

At one point, he had been sitting up in a chair with my husband and kids around him. His hospital gown had become twisted around him, which was making him extremely upset. He asked my husband to help him fix it, and despite my husband's attempts to adjust the gown, he still felt confined by the way it was wrapped around him. So using both hands, he grabbed the reinforced neckline of the gown and ripped it in half. My kids and husband were amazed at the strength he exhibited. Once again, he looked like a man possessed with superhuman strength.

Not only was Dad exhibiting extreme agitation and superhuman strength, but he was also exhibiting poor judgment and shifting boundaries. Dad was always a very respectful, kind man who would never curse in front of a woman or use inappropriate language. At least that was him before he took this medication. I was horrified on a number of occasions through this ordeal to hear Dad cursing at the nurses and making inappropriate advances to them. He asked one nurse to climb into bed with him. I spent a lot of time apologizing to everyone who worked with him at the time and explaining that that was not him. They were all very understanding and claimed that they were not offended. But I felt horrible seeing my father act like this.

This behavior continued into the third day. By this time, I was at my emotional limit. Sam told me to leave the hospital and go take a break. He said he would stay with Dad and let me know if I needed to come back, so I went to Sam's house to feed his dogs and take them for a walk. I was only there for an hour when my phone rang. Sam was calling, and when I answered the phone, in the background, I heard screaming and cursing coming from Dad and pleading coming from the nurses. Sam told me to come back immediately.

When I got back to the hospital, I found four nurses trying to hold Dad down while he was cursing and yelling at them. A doctor came in and gave him an injection that he insisted, once again, would calm him down. Within a little while, he did start to relax. I was not sure if it was due to the medication or the fact that he was becoming completely exhausted. It had been three days of constant tremors and shaking and very little sleep. How long could he endure this?

By the fourth day of this nightmare, I told Dad's doctors that I wanted them to cease all the medications that they were administering. Obviously, nothing that they had tried had helped him. One of the doctors felt that this was not a good decision. He told me that if Dad did not calm down and get some quality sleep very soon, he could die. I was devastated. But since I was Dad's medical power of attorney, I had the power to make medical decisions for him. So after discussing it with Sam, I told the doctors again to stop all medications. And then I began to pray.

I sat by Dad's bed and spoke to him in a calm, soothing voice while I rubbed his head. I told him to take deep breaths and that I was there with him. By the end of that long day, and after all the drugs were out of his system, he finally, mercifully, calmed down and fell asleep for the first time in five days. Sam and I cried tears of relief and joy.

How could his heart and his body have endured this torture for five days? And why did these treatments that were supposed to relax and sedate him, do just the opposite? Could it have something to do with Dad's Alzheimer's disease or his age? Did this class of medication have the opposite effect on people with cognitive issues and older adults?

I decided to search the internet for information on this. What I found was very disturbing. It said that the usual effects of benzodiazepines act similarly to alcohol, causing relaxation and sedation. But that in older adults and in adults with cognitive decline, this class of drugs can cause paradoxical agitation and make them more disinhibited and restless when given these drugs. They can also cause increased confusion, worsening delirium, and accelerated cognitive decline.

I felt so guilty for not researching this earlier and insisting on discontinuing this treatment sooner. Dad had suffered for many days on these medications. I realize that the doctors were trying to help, but my father's case seemed to be very confusing to everyone, and I think that they were trying whatever they could to calm him. However, they should have taken into account his cognitive decline when administering this class of drugs. I had learned a great deal from this experience.

The next day, Dad's doctor informed us that after reviewing the test results, they had determined that he had indeed suffered a stroke. They had consulted with a teaching hospital in Philadelphia, and they had confirmed that even though he did not exhibit the usual symptoms, he had, in fact, had a stroke that left his right side weakened. Because of this, his doctors suggested that he be moved to a rehabilitation hospital to help him regain his strength. They made arrangements to have him transferred in the next few days.

Dad was not pleased about having to go to rehab. But we assured him that it would help to make him strong and independent again. An ambulance transported him from the hospital to rehab. We met with his doctors at the rehab facility who told us about the physical and occupational therapy he would receive. They estimated that he would be there for a few weeks.

We spent the next month watching Dad go through therapy to try to regain his strength. I had requested to have an aide with him around the clock, so when Sam or I could not be there, I felt reassured knowing that there was someone with him at all times.

At one point during Dad's stay at the facility, the nurses had put an adult diaper on him. I was not aware of this when I tried to help him get out of bed to go for a walk. As he pushed himself up out of his bed, he looked down and saw the diaper. He immediately shouted, "What the hell is this? Why am I wearing this?"

I tried to calm him down and divert him from the embarrassment that he was feeling. I pushed the call button for the nurse, and when she arrived, I told her to put underwear on him and to never put a diaper on him again. I remember praying at the time, "Please don't let him ever have to experience this again." I remembered what Dad's doctor had told me after he had administered the Mini-Mental Exam to him: that many people progress to the point of being incontinent. After seeing how upset Dad was at the realization that he was wearing a diaper, how would he ever be able to handle that? And how would I handle seeing my father in that condition? It would be a few more years before I would find out.

When it became obvious that Dad's stay at rehab was going to be longer than what they had originally said, we realized that he would be there over Christmas. We could not have him be there by himself for Christmas, and we were not able to bring him home. So we decided to bring Christmas to him.

I asked at the rehab facility if we could have a private room for the six of us. Not only were they going to give us a private room, but we were going to have access to an oven to warm up the food that we were bringing. We were all set for our Christmas dinner at the rehabilitation hospital.

I cooked the food at home, and we brought everything with us. When we got there, we set everything up in our special, private room. After the food was heated up, we all sat down to our Christmas dinner. It was a very nice day, and Dad was happy.

The next day, I spoke with Dad's doctor to see when he was going to be released. He informed me that, after weeks of physical and occupational therapy, he had not regained the strength that they had hoped for. He told me that Dad was not able to go home and live on his own anymore. He said that either Sam or I should quit our job to be with him all the time or find a facility for him. He also told me that he would be releasing him by the end of the week. My heart dropped. Now what were we going to do?

When Dad was first diagnosed with Alzheimer's disease, Sam and I had visited a number of assisted-living facilities to start getting a feel for them in the event that we needed to place him in one. We visited about ten to twelve facilities and, many times, cried in the parking lot after touring them. We just could not see our father living there. Not only did we not like any of the facilities that we had visited, but most of them had a long waiting list to get in. So when the doctor gave me that news, I knew placing him in an assisted-living home was not going to be an option. I was going to have to give up my job.

I had been working as an Educational Assistant in an elementary school for six years at that time, and I loved my job. It was my escape from the tough situations that I was dealing with in my life. My husband's disability and my father's steady decline were such a heavy burden on my heart. When I went into the school every day and saw the children's smiling, innocent faces, it lifted my spirits and made me forget my troubles for a little while. And when I was able to help a child learn and grow, it gave me the sense of accomplishment that I needed. Since I felt unable to help my husband and father, helping children every day gave me a purpose. I desperately needed that. But my father needed me. So I had a decision to make. That is when divine intervention again came into our lives.

CHAPTER 27

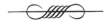

Divine Intervention

S am and I met to try to figure out how we were going to do this. Should we take turns taking Dad to our houses? Sam could not quit his job, so he would get someone to come in during the day to be with Dad until he got home. Dad could stay there for half of the week and then come to my house for half of the week. It sounded like a good plan. Unfortunately, his doctor did not agree.

When we ran this idea by him, he told us that for people with Alzheimer's disease, this type of shuffling around would be very confusing and detrimental. He felt that Dad needed to be in one consistent place. If we were not going to go with a facility, he suggested that Dad stay in his house with around the clock care. The idea sounded wonderful, but where would we find that?

The next day, Sam called me with the strangest story. He was in his kitchen looking out the window, and he saw a lost dog in his yard. He went out to try to check the dog's collar to see if he could find a phone number for the owner when he saw a woman running down the street, yelling, "Malcolm, Malcolm, come Malcolm." Sam took hold of the dog's collar and walked him toward the woman. She was elated to see that Malcolm was okay and thanked Sam profusely.

As they were talking, she introduced herself to Sam. Her name was Patti. Sam asked her where she lived in the neighborhood. She pointed down the street and said that she was currently living at a house where she was the caregiver for a gentleman who had just passed away. However, she told him, she would be moving soon since the gentleman's wife no longer needed assistance. When Sam asked her what she was going to do, she told him she would be looking for another in-home patient to care for. Sam almost fell over in amazement. He told her about Dad and that we were looking for around the clock care for him. She was very excited and said that she would love to help us. He told her he would discuss it with me and get back to her.

When Sam told me about this encounter over the phone, I fell to my knees. If this wasn't divine intervention, I did not know what was. What were the odds of Sam looking out his window at the exact time that Malcolm was in his yard and meeting this caregiver, who just happened to be looking for another patient to care for? It was meant to be.

We made arrangements to meet with Marie, the woman whose husband Patti was taking care of for the past three years. We went to Marie's house when Patti was not there so that we could talk freely. We had a list of questions for her. Was Patti nurturing? Was she dependable? Would she recommend her without any hesitation?

Marie said that Patti had become part of their family in the three years that she had worked for them. Prior to her coming to live with them, she had cared for a friend of theirs for a number of years, and their friend loved her and highly recommended her. Marie said that she was wonderful, caring, dependable, and she would highly recommend her to anyone. We met with Patti, and after giving her a list of our requirements in caring for Dad, we offered her the job. She was very excited and suggested coming to meet with Dad to make sure he was comfortable with her.

We took Patti to the rehab facility, and she immediately gave Dad a hug and introduced herself. She told him that she had a great deal of experience helping elderly patients transition from rehab to home again, and that if he felt comfortable, she would love to help him. He was very agreeable to it, and they seemed to have an instant connection. We left that day feeling like we had won the lottery. Then we realized that we had our work cut out for us.

Since Dad was being released very soon, we needed to get a guest room ready in his house for Patti. We also had to redo the bathroom with grab bars and handicapped accessible items for Dad. Sam called a contractor that he knew who was not busy at the time, and he came over immediately and got to work.

Sam and I went shopping for a bed, dresser, bedding, curtains, and all the things we could think of to make the guest room comfortable for Patti. In three days, we had everything set up and ready. Dad was coming home the next day, and Patti was ready to move in. We just had one problem. There still wasn't a working bathroom.

The contractor had taken the toilet out to fix something, and he did not have everything back together and wouldn't be able to finish it by the next day. Because Dad had a one-bathroom rancher, this was going to create a problem. We asked the rehab facility if they could hold off on Dad's release date, and they said they could not. We were in a panic.

Divine intervention struck again. That night, there was a snowstorm that dumped a foot and a half of snow. The roads were impassable, and there was no way we were going to be able to drive the hour to the rehab facility to pick Dad up. They were going to have to keep him another day. They agreed to this because of the weather conditions. The contractor was able to navigate through the snow and spent the whole day finishing up the bathroom. It was completed by that evening and ready for Dad to come home and Patti to move in the next day. We were so elated.

CHAPTER 28

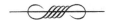

Patti

Patti moved into Dad's house on January 1st. She loved her new room and how warm and welcoming we had made the house for her. We had ordered a new recliner for Dad, and we also purchased one for Patti. I asked her before she moved in what her favorite foods were, and we had stocked the refrigerator with everything that she had mentioned. We were so thankful to have her there caring for our father that we wanted everything to be just perfect for her, and we wanted her to feel at home.

She and Dad had a great connection right from the start. She was very affectionate and nurturing with him, and she made him laugh. We felt so comfortable with her and the attention and care that she was giving him. And he seemed to enjoy her company and feel very at ease with her.

The arrangement was that she would live with Dad and care for him six days a week and would have the day off on Sunday. Sam or I would take Dad on Sunday so that Patti could have the day to herself. We also came to visit a few nights during the week. Barbara and Carla kept their normal schedules of visiting Dad and took him out for walks since Patti did not drive and was not able to get him out. Patti cooked wonderful meals every day and made sure all of Dad's needs were met. He was able to bathe himself and perform some activities of daily living, but Patti was there to make sure he was safe and cared for. She would watch TV with him, do puzzles with him,

145

take him for walks around the neighborhood, and be a companion when we could not be there. She was wonderful.

Life with Patti caring for Dad went very smoothly. I would call every morning to check in. She would give me a detailed report of how he had slept, what he ate for breakfast, and how his spirits were. Then she would put him on the phone, and we would talk for about ten to fifteen minutes. I would repeat this routine at the end of the day, calling to get a report of what he had eaten, what he had done that day, and how he was feeling. Then he and I would talk on the phone for a while. He seemed to be very happy with Patti there, and he seemed to be very well cared for. I would breathe a sigh of relief at the end of every day.

Along with the visits from Barbara, Carla, Sam and I, we also signed Dad up to go to the senior center a few mornings a week. Patti would put him on the senior center bus that came to his house, and he would go to the center to play cards and interact with the other senior citizens that were there. Dad had a very full life and seemed to be very happy with all the accommodations that we had put in place for him.

All these extra activities gave Patti a little break every day since we knew how hard it must have been to be a full-time caregiver. We also did special things for her like giving her gift cards for manicures and pedicures. She was grateful for everything that we did for her. Likewise, we were so appreciative of all that she was doing for us and for Dad.

Summer came, and Patti told us that she wanted to go visit family that she had in Georgia. We had noticed that Patti was starting to look very tired and thin, and I was concerned that caring for Dad was taking a toll on her. I continually asked her if she was okay and if she still felt that she could care for him. She was seventy years old at the time. She assured me that she loved caring for him and that she was fine although a little tired. She felt that this vacation would be good for her. We wholeheartedly agreed that she deserved it.

Sam and I made arrangements to each take Dad to our homes for half of the week. His confusion was gradually getting worse, so he did not understand why he wasn't at his house and where Patti was.

We explained to him that she was away for a little vacation, and he was going to stay with us while she was gone. However, the change in his schedule and routine greatly confused him. While he enjoyed the time with us, he was looking forward to getting back home to his routine and an area that he was familiar with.

We learned over the years of dealing with Alzheimer's disease that when you take the sufferer out of their normal environment, it can be very detrimental to them. Routine and familiarity are a comfort to them in their confused state. Dad definitely exhibited greater confusion and agitation when he stayed with us for the week that Patti was gone.

Patti came back after her week away, still looking tired and run-down. I spoke to her daughter about my concerns, and she assured me that her mother was fine and that she loved caring for Dad. Barbara and Carla also noticed the changes in Patti's appearance and, along with Sam and me, tried to give her more time to rest by taking Dad out more often.

As the summer wound down, I started to notice some very strange behaviors. I would stop in at Dad's house on a hot August afternoon, and all the windows would be closed, and Patti would have a sweater on. When I commented on how hot it was, she said that she was freezing. Dad did not seem to mind the heat, or else I would have insisted that she turn on the air-conditioning, but I thought it was odd that she was so cold on such a warm day.

I also noticed that whenever I took Dad back home after an excursion, Patti was just getting up from a nap. I remember when she first moved in with Dad that she was a very energetic, young seventy-year old woman. But she seemed to be aging before our eyes, and her energy level seemed to be diminishing quickly. She also was becoming thinner by the day.

I approached her at the beginning of September with my concerns and told her that I thought it may be time for us to look for a facility for Dad. Although he had regained his strength from the stroke, he could, in no way, go back to living on his own as his confusion and memory loss were progressing steadily. And I expressed my concerns that caring for him seemed to be taxing on her.

Patti became very upset and said that although she was not feeling like herself, she still needed to work and wanted to continue to care for our father. She said she had grown to love him and did not want to see him go into an assisted-living facility. I agreed to allow her to continue to care for Dad with the promise that she would tell me if it ever became too much for her, and we needed to make other arrangements. She agreed to do this.

September went by without a problem and without any word from Patti that she could not do her job anymore. She continued to look haggard and thin, but we stopped asking her if she was feeling well because it seemed to upset her. I constantly checked in with Dad to see if he was still happy with the arrangement, and he assured me that he was. He was still very well cared for. Everything was going along smoothly. Or so we thought.

Sam called me one afternoon at the beginning of October. He asked if there was any way that I could go stay with Dad that night because Patti had called him and said that she needed to go into the hospital for a few days for some testing. Sam was going out that night and would not be able to do it. I packed a bag and headed to Dad's, wondering what was wrong and why Patti needed to go to the hospital. My calls to her cell phone went unanswered. I prayed that it was nothing serious.

When I got to Dad's, he wasn't able to answer any of my questions about Patti. He said that she seemed fine that day. I told him that she had to go into the hospital for some tests and that I would be staying with him for a few days. I continued to call Patti's cell phone and her daughter's phone to see if she was okay but could not reach anyone.

I made dinner for Dad, and we went for a walk around his neighborhood. After watching TV for a while, Dad went to bed, and I looked around his house to see if there was anything that needed to be done. Patti had left it immaculate like she always did. I found one of her sweaters hanging on the back of a chair in the kitchen and decided to place it in her room. When I went in, I was shocked at what I found.

None of her personal touches were there. The pictures and flower arrangement she kept on the dresser were gone. Her religious statue that she kept on her nightstand was not there. The room felt vacant. I immediately went over to the closet and flung it open. All her clothes were gone! I ran over to the dresser and opened every drawer. Nothing! I remember feeling my heart drop and thinking, "What the hell is going on?"

I immediately called Sam and explained what I had found. I grilled him on what Patti had said to him when she called. He said that she told him that she needed to be admitted to the hospital for a few days, but nothing about moving out. I did not know whether to scream or cry.

I felt betrayed. How could this woman, whom we had trusted with our father and who said that she loved him, do this to us? Why did she just leave and not explain herself? What had happened? My phone calls to her and her daughter remained unanswered. I was awake all that night, trying to figure out what our next steps would be.

The next day, Patti's daughter returned my phone call and gave me some shocking news. Apparently, her mother had had cancer for a while and did not want anyone to know. Because she needed to continue to work, she withheld this information from us because she was afraid that we would either find another caregiver or place Dad in a facility. She was hoping to keep working for as long as she could.

I felt a combination of sympathy for Patti and her condition and betrayal at her not being honest with us and leaving us stranded with no one to care for Dad. I had asked her repeatedly if she was feeling well and if the strain of caring for Dad was too much for her. And she continuously assured me that she was feeling fine and that she would let me know if she felt that she could no longer handle it. I was extremely angry with her and her lack of honesty. However, the sympathy overtook the anger, and I told her daughter to please tell Patti that we were praying for her and that we loved her.

Patti died a week after she left Dad's house. When her daughter called to tell me, I was shocked and saddened that she had been so sick and continued to work under those conditions. She truly was trying to work as long as she could.

I went through another roller-coaster ride of emotions that day. Sadness over the loss of Patti and how she must have suffered, a lingering feeling of betrayal that she was not honest with us, and panic over what we were going to do about Dad's care. We had the next few days covered. Sam and I were going to take turns staying with him, and Barbara and Carla would be there to assist when we needed them. But what were we going to do long term? It was time to find a facility for Dad to live in that could give him twenty-four-hour care. I realized that we had to start looking for a place. I prayed for divine intervention to step in again. My prayers were answered.

CHAPTER 29

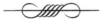

Briarwood

Sam and I made a list of all the assisted-living facilities that we had looked at when Dad was first diagnosed, as well as a few new ones that we had researched. I dreaded this because of what I remembered from our initial search years ago. There were many places that we had visited that made me feel physically ill. How were we going to put our father into one of these facilities?

One of the first things that I noticed about many of these places was the odor. Many times, we would be greeted with the strong stench of urine the minute that we walked in the door. Sam and I would look at each other and immediately turn around and walk out.

Another feature that we noticed about many of the facilities that we visited was the drabness of the lobby. First impressions are everything. If the lobby was the first thing that a visitor saw when they walked in, and it did not look appealing and welcoming, what did the rest of the place look like? We knew from our previous tours that many of these facilities had long waiting lists to get in, so we knew we had to get started right away. I took a few days off from work, and we set out on our search with a feeling of dread.

The first place that we visited was one that had gotten rave reviews both from people that we knew and from online research. We walked in and asked to talk to their executive director. A few minutes later, we were sitting in her office, and I started crying.

I explained our situation and that we needed to find assisted-living for our father. I inquired about their waiting list and if there was any way to admit him as soon as possible. She began asking us questions about Dad's abilities.

"Is your father still able to feed himself?" she asked.

Sam and I looked at each other in bewilderment. "Yes," we both replied.

"Is he still able to dress himself?"

Again, we answered affirmatively.

"Your father is not ready for our facility," she informed us. "We are more of a nursing home and skilled-care facility. I think your father would do well at Briarwood."

I looked at the list that was on my lap. Briarwood was not listed on it.

"Where is Briarwood?" I asked her.

"It's right around the corner from here. It's a wonderful facility, and I happen to know the executive director there. Go over and ask for Cathy Quinley and tell her that I sent you," she said.

I was so excited that I wanted to hug her.

We left there and drove to Briarwood. When we pulled up to the building, we were amazed to see what looked like a luxury hotel. And when we walked into the lobby, we were greeted with a beautiful baby grand piano with a huge arrangement of fresh flowers on top of it. We were also pleasantly surprised at the soft music playing and the wonderful aroma of flowers and something delicious cooking.

I walked up to the smiling, friendly receptionist and asked for Cathy Quinley.

"I'm sorry," she said. "Do you have an appointment?"

"No," I replied. "We just came from another facility, and they recommended we come here and speak to Cathy."

"Well, you will have to come back at another time because she is in a meeting," she replied.

We were very disappointed. We knew this was too good to be true. We thanked the receptionist and began to walk toward the exit. Suddenly she called out to us and said, "Wait a minute, I think she just got back from her meeting. Let me check."

We waited while she made a phone call, and when she hung up, she told us to go right into Cathy's office. Cathy greeted us, and we immediately told her who had sent us to see her. She responded with an enormous smile on her face and said that she would take care of us. Once again, I started to cry. I explained our situation and asked if there was any way that Dad could be placed on a waiting list there. And she smiled.

"I happen to have a room that just opened up. It is on the second floor right off the elevator and right near our activities room. It is one of the best rooms we have with regards to the location."

Sam and I looked at each other and smiled through our tears.

Cathy took us up to look at the room, and we could not have been more elated. It was a sun-filled, beautiful room that was, in fact, perfectly stationed near the activities room and the tables where all the residents on that floor gathered at night to play cards and games. This room was perfect for Dad. And it had just opened up. Divine intervention had struck again!

Now we had to figure out if Dad had the money to cover the monthly cost. I told Cathy what he earned every month from his pension, social security, and veteran's benefits, and we were ecstatic to find out that it would cover the cost of the room. We signed the papers that day, and Cathy assured me that the room would be painted and cleaned in a few days. We could move Dad into his new residence in less than a week.

We walked out to the parking lot, and Sam and I cried and hugged each other. Someone had truly been looking out for us. This could not have worked out more perfectly. Then we both stopped and looked at each other with a look of fear. What if Dad did not want to come here? How were we going to convince him? What were we going to tell him?

At this point in Dad's disease progression, he had no concept of time. He confused morning and evening, seasons, and length of time. He and I would be out to dinner, and the sun would very clearly be setting, and he would reply, "Wow, it's a beautiful morning." Or we would get ready to leave his house for a walk on a hot day in the summer, and he would go to the closet to get his winter coat.

Length of time was also a problem. I would have just left his house after visiting all day, and Sam would call Dad and say, "Did you have a nice day with Maryanne today?"

And Dad would reply, "No, I haven't seen her in a while. She must be away on vacation."

So Sam and I decided to use this deficit to our advantage.

Barbara had been staying with Dad while Sam and I were on our search. When we got to his house, we told Barbara of our plan, and we all agreed that it just might work. After she left, we sat Dad down and told him what we needed to do.

We had not told him about Patti's death as we did not want to upset him, and we were not sure he would understand. So we just told him that Patti was not feeling well and had to go into the hospital for a few weeks. We said that Sam and I both had to work, so we would not be able to care for him during the day. Because of this, we were going to move him into an apartment for veterans temporarily until Patti came back. We told him that all expenses would be taken care of because he was a veteran—the rent, all his meals, and all housekeeping fees. Of course, this was not true, but we thought it would help Dad if he thought he was being rewarded for being a veteran.

Dad was very proud of his military background. He fought for his country and, as a result, felt that he was entitled to any benefits that were given to veterans. He took advantage of the GI Bill after being honorably discharged from World War II and went to school to become a welder. He received a monthly veterans allowance for being wounded while in the war. And he visited the veterans hospital to receive care. So when he heard that he was going to be able to live somewhere completely free because of his veteran's status, he was agreeable to the new arrangement. He felt like he was being repaid for serving his country. We felt awful lying to him, but we needed all the help we could get in getting Dad to go along with this transition. And if he knew how much assisted-living facilities cost, he would have balked at the idea of spending all that money.

We spent the next week making plans for moving Dad's furniture and clothes into his new "apartment." We did not want him to see us packing since he thought he was only going for a few days, so we decided to have Carla take him out for the day while we packed up his things and moved them over to Briarwood. She planned to drop him off there in a few hours, and we would have everything set up. We prayed that Dad's memory failure would pay off this time when he got there and saw his furniture in the apartment. We hoped we could pass it off as a furnished apartment with furniture that just happened to resemble his own.

When Carla brought Dad to his new apartment, he was very pleased. He liked the coziness of the room and how bright it was due to the large windows that allowed the sun in. He never commented on the furniture, which we were so thankful for. So far so good. Now we had to try to get him involved socially.

As I said, the location of his room could not have been more perfect. Right outside his door was a lobby with five or six tables with comfortable chairs surrounding all of them. Many of the residents on his floor, as well as residents on the first floor, gathered here at night to play cards or just talk. And a few steps further down the hall was a large entertainment room. This is where they held shows, played bingo, had sing-alongs, and gathered for all holiday parties that the facility held. I was so excited and felt that the location of his room was going to be ideal for Dad.

Sam and I decided to take turns staying with him for the first few nights to help him get adjusted. Sam stayed the first night, and Dad seemed fine. But when I arrived there the second evening, while many people were gathered at the tables outside his door, laughing and talking, he was in his room with the door closed. When I walked in and asked him why he was not out with the other residents, he stated that he did not know any of them and wanted to stay in his room. I was very upset.

I went out into the lobby and was greeted by a wonderful, kindly woman named Anna. She smiled and introduced herself to me. When she asked me why I looked so upset, I told her about my father being new to Briarwood and my worries about him not getting involved and meeting people. She immediately eased my worries.

"Don't you worry about anything, honey," she said. "I'll take care of your dad and make sure he gets involved in everything. I'm very active here, and I will make sure he doesn't stay in his room." She then got up, went to Dad's room, knocked on the door, and went in and introduced herself. Then, in no uncertain terms, she told him that he was not going to sit in his room every night. He was going to come out and play cards with her and her friends.

Dad laughed and said, "Okay, that sounds good to me." That was the start of a beautiful friendship.

Anna became my eyes and ears at Briarwood. She would tell me if there was something going on with Dad that she felt that I needed to be aware of. She became his social director, his friend, his confidante. And she became a member of our family of caregivers for Dad.

There wasn't a time that I went to visit Dad that Anna was not sitting next to him at a sing-along or a show. Or that they weren't playing bingo or Wii together, along with a group of other residents. She said that he reminded her of her father, and she grew to love him. And we grew to love her.

Unfortunately, Anna's family did not come to visit her, and she was very lonely. So we took her under our wing. Whenever we visited Dad, we also visited with Anna. Whenever I went to the store to buy something for Dad, I bought something for Anna. I could never repay her for the peace of mind that she gave me, knowing that my father was being "watched over" by someone when we were not there.

The transition to Briarwood went very smoothly. Dad, at first, asked when he was going to go home. We told him that Patti needed to stay in the hospital for a while and that he was going to be staying at his new apartment until she got better. As I said, he no longer had any concept of time. So we were able to tell him this until he got used to his new surroundings. Then he forgot about his home, and Briarwood became his new normal as well as our new normal.

CHAPTER 30

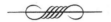

Life at Briarwood

All my concerns about Dad adjusting to Briarwood were laid to rest as time went on. He seemed to like his cozy room, he was eating three delicious, healthy meals a day, and he participated in many social activities. I felt relief with the arrangements that we had made for his care.

Along with Sam and I, Dad still continued to receive visits every week from Barbara and Carla, which made him very happy. It also made him the envy of many of the other residents there. Countless people who lived there never received a visitor, which was so sad to see. Some of them would stop me and tell me that I was such a good daughter for coming to see my father. They would go on to tell me that their children never came to visit them. I did not know whether to believe their stories or not because many of them suffered from Alzheimer's disease like Dad, and I thought that perhaps they just did not remember their children's visits. However, over the more than two years that Dad lived there, Briarwood held numerous family picnics, holiday dinners, and dances that the resident's families were invited to. Many of them had no family members show up. We always tried to include these residents at our table.

Unfortunately, this is something that is prevalent in these facilities. Many of the nurses and aides that worked at Briarwood told me that a large population of the residents were basically dropped off there and forgotten about by their families. This broke my heart.

How could you do this to a parent or other loved one? Just seeing the way their faces would light up when I would say hello to them or ask them about their day made me realize just how much they craved attention. While the nurses and aides were wonderful, there was no substitution for the love and attention from family.

Sam and I tried to help some of these people as much as we could. Whenever we would take Dad on his weekly trip to the grocery store to pick up his favorite snacks, one or two of the residents would ask us to pick up something for them and tell us they would reimburse us when we got back. Invariably, by the time we got back with whatever it was that they needed, they would forget about reimbursement. We didn't care—we just felt good about helping these people who had obviously been forgotten by their families.

True to her word, Anna always made sure that she watched out for Dad and reported anything to me that she felt I should be aware of. As I said, Anna was one of the residents whose children never came to see her, so I, in return, always made sure to look out for her and include her in our family visits. I also included her requests on my shopping list whenever I went to the store. This worked out well for the most part, except for the time that she asked me to pick up a bottle of wine and new bras for her! I got the bras, but made excuses for not getting her the wine. I wasn't sure if that was something that her doctor would approve of.

Over Dad's time at Briarwood, there were a myriad of fun activities that he participated in. All these activities were good for him cognitively. At the sing-alongs, he would remember words to old songs that he knew. Studies show that Alzheimer's disease patients respond well to music stimulation, and we found this to be true with Dad. While he could not remember names or places or if he had eaten dinner, he would always remember words to songs and sing along and clap his hands. Music was truly beneficial to him, and I would highly recommend it for anyone suffering from Alzheimer's disease. Bingo was another activity that was very advantageous for Dad. It would force him to use his mind in recognizing the letters and numbers that were called. Playing cards, again, allowed him to use his thinking and communication skills. All these activities are so beneficial to someone with Alzheimer's disease and were stimulations that he was not afforded when he lived alone. For this reason, I was so happy that we had moved Dad into this facility. This is something that is very important to consider when moving a loved one to an assisted-living facility for cognitive decline. What will they do to stimulate them mentally and socially? I was happy to see that Briarwood was fulfilling this requirement.

Some of the activities that Briarwood held were so entertaining that I could not wait to attend them myself. There was a Western barbecue in the spring, in which the staff all dressed in cowboy boots and hats, and we had ribs and baked beans. Once, when I was visiting, they had an Elvis impersonator that I enjoyed so much that I missed an appointment that I had needed to get to. Dad thoroughly enjoyed it also, except that he thought that it really was Elvis Presley performing. Unfortunately, this was when I was still correcting him, and I had to inform him that Elvis had died and that this was someone just imitating him. He was shocked to learn that the king had died, but we still enjoyed the show.

Each year at Christmas, Briarwood held a family Christmas dinner that was absolutely amazing. The whole facility was decorated beautifully, and there was a Santa Claus there who went around to speak to all the residents. The food was delicious, and there were gifts for everyone. It was a very special event that brought a smile to everyone's face. All these activities and special events brought such joy and happiness to the people living at Briarwood. This is a very important part of any facility, as it lends to the quality of life of its residents.

One of the aspects that I learned about with Dad's assisted-living facility, and I'm sure it is true in other facilities, is that the squeaky wheel gets the grease. The people whose children did not visit and check up on things were not as well taken care of as Dad was. Their rooms were not as clean, their hygiene was not as good, and there was not the attention to detail that Dad was receiving. Of course, I was a very loud, squeaky wheel.

Whenever I visited Dad, I had a checklist of items that I scrutinized. I also made sure that whoever else visited him went through the list and reported back to me if anything was wrong. Was his hair brushed? Were his dentures in? Were his clothes and room clean?—These were all the things that I expected Briarwood to make sure were done. Because we were there on a regular basis, and not always on a set schedule, these stipulations were always fulfilled the way we expected them to be. These impromptu, frequent visits ensured that Dad received that little extra care. And it helped to keep the facility on their toes.

One particular requirement that I had to stay on top of was the delivery of Dad's daily newspaper. Before he moved to Briarwood, his morning routine would involve going outside to get his newspaper and then reading it from cover to cover while drinking his coffee. His paper was always delivered at the end of his driveway. As his memory started to decline, I was worried about him walking to the end of the driveway and, perhaps, not being able to find his way back. So I called and asked if they could deliver it to his front door, which they did. He just had to open the door and get the newspaper.

Reading the newspaper was very beneficial to Dad. Sometimes he would be able to recall something that he had read, and he would tell me about it. It also filled his morning. As his disease progressed, it would sometimes fill his whole day. I watched him on one occasion as he read an article on the front page. When it came time to continue the article on page 8, he turned to that page. When he finished the article, he returned to the front page and began the article again. He would get stuck in a continuous loop. But it kept him occupied, and he was using his brain, which was so important. That is why I wanted this morning routine to continue for Dad at Briarwood.

When he moved in, I had his subscription transferred. However, they could only deliver the newspaper to the front desk, not to Dad's second-floor room. I knew that he would not remember to go to the front desk to pick it up, so the people at Briarwood assured me that someone would bring the newspaper to Dad in the morning or give it to him when he came down for breakfast. I felt relieved. The plan worked for a while. But as time went on, it became time to start squeaking.

I called Dad every morning before I went to work to see how he was feeling, how he had slept, and just to say hello. I also asked him if he was reading his newspaper. Many mornings, he told me that he did not have it. So I would hang up the phone and call the front desk. I would very nicely ask if his newspaper was there, and they would tell me that it was and then assure me that someone would run it right up to him. I would thank them and wait about twenty minutes. Then I would call Dad again.

"Hi, Dad. Did you get your newspaper?," I would inquire. Sometimes he responded that he did, and sometimes he said he did not. So on the occasions that he did not, I would call the front desk again. This happened off and on for about a month. Many times, my phone calls were not quite as nice, I'm sorry to say. But it finally got resolved, and Dad received his newspaper every morning. I think they were tired of hearing from me!

As I said, for the most part, Briarwood took care of everything to our satisfaction. There were not too many incidents that I had to get combative about. But one particular incident caused quite a stir and ended up benefitting all the residents.

As Dad's disease progressed and he became more incontinent, the director consulted with me about having him wear "adult underwear." She was careful not to use the term "diaper" as she knew how sensitive I was to the idea of my father wearing a diaper. She felt that he should at least wear one at night in the event that he had an accident. I agreed to this along with her suggestion that I get a waterproof mattress pad for his bed. I had noticed that some of the resident's rooms smelled of stale urine, and I suspected that it had to do with incontinent issues and accidents that had happened in bed and on the furniture. We had bought Dad a new mattress when he had moved to Briarwood, so the waterproof pad was a great idea. I went out that day and bought two of them and put Dad's name on them in permanent marker. On my next visit, I put his new mattress pad on his bed and put the spare one in the drawer to be used when housekeeping washed the other one. I was happy with this new plan.

A few weeks later, Katelyn and I were visiting with Dad when I noticed an odor in his room. I started following my nose and ended up at his bed. The bed was made, so I pulled the comforter back to inspect. What greeted me caused my blood to boil. His sheets were soaking wet with urine, and when I pulled the fitted sheet off, the waterproof pad was not there. There was a huge wet spot on the mattress and a stain that indicated that it had been wet before and had dried.

The scene that took place after my discovery is not something that I am proud of, but I could not help myself. I ran angrily down the hall yelling for the nurses and aides to get the director up to my father's room immediately. I also demanded that housekeeping get there right away with something to clean Dad's mattress. My poor daughter was practically hiding from the embarrassment that her mother was causing her, but I was out of control. All that I kept thinking about was that if we had not been there that day, Dad would have gotten into a urine saturated bed when he went to sleep that night.

How many nights had that already happened? Wasn't this what we were trying to avoid when the director convinced me to put Dad in adult underwear and to get waterproof mattress pads for his bed? Where was the pad that I had put on his bed? And where was the spare one that I noticed was no longer in his drawer? Who was the incompetent person who had made Dad's bed without checking to make sure that he had not had an accident? These were all the questions that I was firing at the director when she came flying into Dad's room a few minutes later.

She had no answers. She asked housekeeping about the mattress pads, but no one knew where they were. She assured me that she would find out who had made the bed without checking it and speak to them. And she had staff from housekeeping scrub Dad's mattress with bleach to get it clean until we could get him a new one, which she said she would reimburse us for.

After I had calmed down and could speak rationally, I suggested that they needed to put a new policy in place with regards to this issue. How many other residents was this happening to? Is this why some of their rooms smelled so bad? I suggested that she make it a policy with housekeeping that they inspect each resident's bed before making it in the morning. And that it should be mandatory that each resident's bed have a waterproof pad on it.

A month later, the director informed me that they had ordered waterproof pads for each resident, and it was now standard that each bed be made with these on them. Also, the morning routine for housekeeping was that they pull the bedding back and inspect the mattress before making the bed. She thanked me for bringing this to her attention and assured me that this would never happen again. So while my tirade was a little extreme, I felt that I had made a difference for all the residents at Briarwood. From that time on, Dad's bed was always clean, and there was never a foul odor in his room.

I would recommend to anyone whose loved one is in an assisted-living or care facility to make sure you stay on top of their care. Let them know your expectations, stop in at all different times unexpectedly, and speak up when things are not done the way you want them done. You need to advocate for your loved one because, in many cases, they cannot advocate for themselves. The squeaky wheel truly does get the grease.

CHAPTER 31

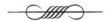

Making Adjustments

With each step in the Alzheimer's disease progression, we found that we had to make many adjustments for Dad. There were many things that he was no longer able to do. We were trying so hard to make him still feel independent, so it required us to find ways to accommodate his declining abilities.

One area that we noticed he was having trouble with was using his remote control for his television. I arrived at Briarwood many times to find the television unplugged from the wall. When I asked Dad why he unplugged it, he told me that he didn't. However, I was with him one evening, and as we were leaving for dinner, he went to the wall and unplugged the TV to turn it off. I asked him if he knew how to use the remote control, and he said, "Of course I do." But I was certain that he did not know how.

At the time, Dad had a remote control with more buttons than he had ever used. I sometimes had trouble figuring out my own remote control so, of course, he was having trouble. I set out to find a simple one with only a few buttons on it.

I searched the internet and found the perfect one. It had an "ON" button, an "OFF" button, and two buttons with arrows up and down for the volume and the channels. This was perfect for Dad. I ordered it online and could not wait to show him his new, simpler remote.

When it arrived, I showed him how much easier it was to use with only the four buttons that he would need. He was excited about it, and I felt relieved that he would no longer have to unplug the TV every time he wanted to turn it off.

One evening, I was on the phone with Dad, and he could not hear me because his television was too loud.

I said, "Dad, turn the TV down so that you can hear what I'm saying."

He replied, "How do I do that?"

I told him to pick up the remote control on his coffee table and push the volume button down.

"What remote control?" he asked.

I replied, "It's the little plastic thing on your coffee table, Dad."

I heard him pick it up, and he said, "There is no volume button on this thing."

I said, "Dad, there should be an ON button, an OFF button, and two arrow buttons for the volume and channel."

He insisted that it had none of those buttons on it. When I asked him to read to me what was on his "remote," he said, "It says Ice Breakers Mints."

He had picked up the plastic container of mints that was on his coffee table instead of the remote control. Obviously, working the television was getting to be too difficult for him. He went back to just unplugging the TV whenever he was finished watching it.

Another adjustment that we had to make was with Dad's clothes. He had always worn button-down shirts, long sleeved in the winter, and short sleeved in the summer. And they always had a pocket for his reading glasses. However, he was now having trouble buttoning his shirts. Many times, when I would arrive, a few of the buttons were left undone, or they were done incorrectly. I would fix it for him and make a joke about it so as not to embarrass him. But I realized that this was becoming an issue for him, so I set out to buy him new shirts with no buttons. Of course, they had to have a pocket for his glasses though.

Next was his sneakers. I noticed one day that Dad was having trouble tying them. At times, he was able to do it, but it was an extremely slow process. And at other times, he would just look at his shoes and not have any idea where to start. So I went out in search of sneakers with Velcro on them. This was an enormous help to him, and he seemed to adjust to this change well.

Along with Dad no longer being able to button his shirts or tie his shoes, he also could no longer figure out how to put on a seat belt. Every time he got into my car to go on one of our outings, I would have to remind him to put his seat belt on. He would reach over his shoulder for it but then have no idea what to snap it into. There were times that he tried to snap it into the dashboard, the gear shift, and once into my water bottle that was in the cup holder. Ever trying not to have him lose his dignity, I would show him where it needed to go and then hope that he could do it himself. However, there were many times that I had to buckle him in, much like I had to buckle my children in when they were babies. There were many times that I was rendered speechless as I thought to myself that this man could take a car apart and put it back together before Alzheimer's disease, and now he could not figure out how to handle a seat belt.

After Dad's stroke, his balance became an issue. Whereas before the stroke he was able to walk perfectly without any issues, he was now stumbling at times and more hunched over than he had been. At the doctor's suggestion, we purchased a rollator walker for him. This was a walker with four wheels and a built-in seat so that he could sit if he got tired. It was an ideal solution for Dad's balance issues. Or so we thought.

One of the major issues that Alzheimer's disease sufferers have is the inability to learn anything new. As was the case with Dad's hearing aids and the cell phone that we had gotten him, this new walker was something foreign to him. He had never used an assistive device in his life, and learning how to use this new item was a challenge. A challenge that led to many repetitive conversations.

Whenever Dad would get up to start walking, I would put the walker in front of him and remind him to use it. Undoubtedly, he would say, "What is this?"

I would explain that it was his "new" walker (this conversation was still happening a year after he had started using it, so it was no longer new), and that his doctor wanted him to use it so that he would not fall. He would agree, walk with it to our next destination, sit down, and then the whole process would start over again when he would go to stand up. Many times, when we were in the grocery story, and I would go to put the cart away in the corral, Dad would put his walker there, thinking that it belonged to the store. His walker was a huge area of frustration for both he and I. For him, it was frustrating because he had never used a walker and could not understand why he needed one now. And, for me, because explaining it to him so many times during the course of a visit made me want to pull my hair out!

Due to the fact that an Alzheimer's patient's abilities to do simple activities of daily living are declining every day, it is very important to find items to help them retain as much independence and dignity as they can. It is also important to realize that these new items may take them some time to get used to. Or because of their inability to learn new things, they may never get used to them. In that case, take deep breaths and get ready to explain it to them repeatedly.

CHAPTER 32

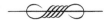

Caregiver Burnout

Caring for anyone with a mental or physical disability is extremely taxing. Many times, the caregivers themselves start to suffer mental and physical ailments due to the stress of this difficult job and the devastating toll that it takes on them. Compared with caregivers of people without Alzheimer's disease, twice as many caregivers of those with the disease indicate substantial emotional, financial, and physical difficulties. Due to the constant worry and duties that go with this job, it is not uncommon to see a person in this role require medical or psychological care themselves. It is very important to realize when to reach out for this care.

I found myself, over the long course of Dad's illness, with many maladies that I needed help with. One of the most severe of these was depression. There were days that I did not want to get out of bed, days that all I wanted to do was cry and curl up in a ball. I realized that I needed help.

I decided to research what I was feeling to see if I was losing my mind. I googled "Caregiver Burnout" and found many sites that listed the symptoms of it. I was shocked at how many of them I exhibited. Some of the symptoms were the following:

- Withdrawal from friends and family
- Loss of interest in activities previously enjoyed
- Feeling blue, irritable, hopeless, and helpless

- Changes in appetite, weight, or both
- Changes in sleep patterns
- Getting sick more often
- Feelings of wanting to hurt yourself or the person for whom you are caring
- Emotional and physical exhaustion
- Excessive use of alcohol and/or sleep medications
- Irritability

I had definitely withdrawn from people, lost interest in activities, felt hopeless and helpless, could not eat or sleep, was exhausted most of the time, was very irritable, and drank a lot. Yes, I had caregiver burnout.

I spoke to my doctor about Dad's illness and what I was experiencing as his caregiver. I told her about my feelings of despair and inability to cope. She suggested an Alzheimer's support group. She also thought that I should try an antidepressant. I was very receptive to both ideas.

I started my antidepressant immediately and began to seek out a support group. I contacted the Alzheimer's Association to see if there was one in my area. I asked Sam if he would like to attend with me, and he said he wanted to. So we began to attend a group together.

While I feel that support groups can be very beneficial, Sam and I did not feel that we could relate to the other members of this particular one as they were all spouses of people with Alzheimer's disease. And they were all much older than us. There were no other members of the group who were our age and dealing with a parent with Alzheimer's. Sam and I were forty-six and fifty, respectively, and Dad was ninety-one at the time. Most of our peer's parents were much younger and still relatively healthy. So we could not relate to the people who were in the group. While the feelings of desperation and helplessness were the same, the logistics of juggling a family, a job, and caregiving were not. We attended a few sessions and then stopped going.

My family doctor suggested a therapist. So I found one in my area and began seeing her twice a week. These sessions were filled with many tears, both on my part and the therapist's. One day, as I described my feelings of complete and utter despair in trying to care for my father, my husband, and my two teenagers, we both reached for the tissue box that she kept on her coffee table at the same time. She genuinely felt my pain and was supportive and helpful as I fought my way through the depression and anguish. I continued to see her until my dad passed away. I would highly recommend therapy to anyone dealing with caregiver burnout.

One of the most important things that a caregiver for someone who is ill will find out, and that I discovered while going through this eight-year battle, was who is there to support you along the way. You do not really know the character of the people in your lives until you experience a tragedy. That is when their true colors come out.

I can honestly say that my husband was my lifeline. My poor husband lived with the despair every day as I cried, screamed, and fought my way through the burnout that I was feeling. He hung in there when I was numb with sadness and still tried to make me laugh and smile when it was close to impossible for me. The vows "for better or for worse" were truly tested in our marriage as I was at my worst, many times taking out my frustration on him. While he did not precisely understand what I was going through as he had never experienced it with anyone in his family, he loved my father and felt the pain along with me of seeing him decline sharply. I will be forever thankful to my husband for the love and support that he showed me through this grueling time of my life.

Next were my children. My poor children went through eight years of not having a mother that was truly present in their lives. While I may have been physically there, there were many times when my mind was not on what they were saying or doing. And they could tell. But they knew that I had to care for their grandfather, and they were understanding and supportive through it all. And in the later years of the disease, they both chipped in and helped with his care. I am so grateful for my children and impressed by their character in tough situations.

Then there was my partner in all this, my brother. We were truly a team for the eight years that we struggled through this disease.

I don't know that I would have been able to do what I did had my brother not been along for the ride with me. We split the duties, we cried together, we vented to each other, and we leaned on each other through the whole ordeal. I felt incredibly lucky to have Sam by my side throughout this roller-coaster ride and saw the true character of my brother in how he cared for our father.

I have had many friends throughout my life. And I have also lost many friends. One of my best friends, who was my maid of honor in my wedding, comes to mind as one of the friends I have lost. I consider her a fair-weather friend. Fair-weather friends are people who are there with you through the good times, to laugh and enjoy life and coast along with you when things are going great. But should a tragedy arise, they are nowhere to be found.

After my mother died, I spent basically every day for the first few months crying. This friend would call to check up on me from time to time, but I could tell she did not know what to say or do when I would break down. One day, a few months after my mother's death, this friend told me that she could no longer speak to me because I was making her very depressed every time that we spoke. I was shocked. I had thought that a true friend would stick by my side through the good times as well as the bad. Needless to say, we never spoke again after that conversation.

I began to gauge my relationships with people based on the criteria of whether or not they would be there for me "for better or for worse." Many people who should have been there to support me, people whom I had supported in the past, were not there for me. So throughout the many trials and tribulations I have had in my life, I have written off many people.

However, during the course of my dad's long illness, I honestly found out who my friends are. And I had many incredible ones who were there with me every step of the journey. Each phone conversation, each dinner date, each outing with my friends would consist of my litany of complaints about Dad's decline. Many of these conversations would involve me crying, and these wonderful people having to console me repeatedly. But they hung in there with me over the many years and gave me constant support and encouragement. They were truly better than any therapist that I had seen or any support group that I had attended. I felt so blessed to have these remarkable people in my life.

While I clearly exhibited many of the signs of caregiver burn-out, I was able to recognize that I needed help. My antidepressants definitely helped with my mood fluctuations. Seeking out a support group gave me the sense of not being alone in this battle. Seeing a therapist allowed me to get my feelings out with someone who was neutral and nonjudgmental. And most importantly, I was fortunate to have a tremendous support system. My family and friends kept me afloat when I thought I would drown under the burden of care-giving. I will be forever grateful to all of them for being there for me through this challenging time in my life.

CHAPTER 33

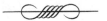

Irrational Feelings

There were so many times during Dad's illness that I experienced thoughts that I was embarrassed to admit to. The frustration at having to explain things repeatedly to him, the loss of patience when he would repeat the same thing for about the twentieth time in as many minutes, and the prayers that he would just pass away peacefully so that we would not have to see the end stage of the disease were just some of these thoughts. In all the research that I did, I learned that these were all perfectly normal emotions when dealing with this debilitating, long illness. However, the one emotion that I could not understand was anger. I was very angry with my father.

While I did not experience this emotion continuously throughout the entire eight years of his decline, there were times that I looked at him and did not see the man that I had grown up with, and I was angry at him for that. Then I would get angry at myself for being angry at him. What the heck was going on?

When my husband suffered his spinal cord injury in 2009, my children were incredible. They helped in any way that they could, they were supportive to both me and their father, and they seemed to adjust to our new way of life rather well. My husband was no longer able to do the things that they had always seen him do, like cut the grass, wash the cars, or just go for a walk. I was so busy just trying to take care of everyone and keep some sense of normalcy that I did not really notice any change in either of them. I was proud of how strong they were being.

A few years after my husband's injury, it became obvious that, while he had made some significant progress, he was not going to be the man that my children were used to. Walking was difficult for him, and he needed crutches at all times. He was tired a majority of the time due to the struggles that he had with walking, and he was no longer able to work, which affected him mentally. We had to accept that this was our new normal.

At this time, Katelyn was eighteen and dealing with her own life changes. She had graduated high school and decided to do her first two years of college at a Penn State campus close to home and commute. While she was living at home with us, there were times that she was extremely agitated and angry. I chalked this up to her first year of college and the transition that she was experiencing with that. However, I also noticed that she was not very kind to her father. He would ask her to do things for him, and she would huff and puff and roll her eyes and eventually do what he had asked, but definitely not willingly.

After observing this for quite some time, I decided to discuss this behavior with her. What she told me was extremely eye-opening. She said that she was angry with her dad for not being the same. She knew that this was not a rational thought, but she could not help it. She looked at him and did not see the same father that she had grown up with. And she was angry with him for that.

It was like a bolt of lightning had hit me. I sat there in aston-ishment as I made the connection to how I was feeling with my own father. The man that had always been there for me, caring for me and protecting me, was no longer that man. He now needed my care, and he was never going to be the same. And I was angry about that, just like Katelyn was with her dad. Was this a normal way to feel? Time to do some research again.

I googled, "Is it normal to be angry at someone who is sick?" Up popped many articles that I devoured. One article by Dr. Laura Sills, a licensed clinical psychologist, stated that feeling angry at someone who is sick was a typical reaction. She states, "When we are around someone we love who is significantly emotionally or physically impaired due to chronic or acute illness and we cannot make the problem go away or stop our loved one's suffering, it is very frustrating. Watching helplessly as someone you love suffers makes us suffer, too. It is this pain that we get angry about and can easily take out on the one who is ill. Without realizing it, we may show great intolerance to and irritation with a person's limitations when they are sick."

Another article by Kate Harveston, a health and healthcare journalist, claimed that "you may feel guilty for being angry at someone who is suffering. But, if you're wondering if you can feel both compassion and anger at someone suffering from an illness, the answer is yes." She went on to say that you need to understand that you are a human being experiencing human reactions, and you need to channel your emotions in healthy ways.

Many of the articles that I read talked about self-help and not being equipped to care for others if you did not take care of yourself first. They stressed eating healthy, getting plenty of exercise and sleep, and finding time in your day to just release your feelings. One article in particular made me feel normal when I truly felt that I had lost my mind.

An article by Dr. Paul Haider, a spiritual teacher, stated that to release your feelings of anger you could go outside and throw rocks against a wall, scream into your pillow, or scream in your car at night. How did Dr. Haider know that I had done that? There was one night, in particular, that came to mind while reading this article. I had been driving home from seeing Dad and felt that I was losing my grip on sanity. So I began screaming. And screaming. And screaming. I was literally driving down a dark road at night, screaming at the top of my lungs. When I finally stopped, I thought that I had definitely crossed over the line of sanity. But to my surprise, I felt better! I felt lighter. And I actually laughed at myself. I had released the angry feelings, and it felt so good and therapeutic.

Katelyn got over the anger that she felt toward her father, and they have a terrific relationship today. She truly respects the wonderful man that he is and no longer sees his disability. Now when he asks her to do something for him, there is no longer anger and resentment. She loves him wholeheartedly.

During the years of my father's decline, I was able to put my anger at the disease in perspective and appreciate the wonderful man that he was. I am still angry at Alzheimer's disease for what it did to him. But I have come to realize that the irrational feelings that I was experiencing were normal, human feelings that are felt when you are watching someone you love change before your eyes, and there is nothing that you can do to stop it. The only thing that you can do is love them unconditionally.

CHAPTER 34

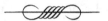

The Alzheimer's Unit

One morning, in early September of 2013, I received a disturbing phone call from Randy, the director of Briarwood. She informed me that they were going to have to move Dad from the assisted-living section of the facility to the Alzheimer's unit. She felt that he had advanced to the severe stages of Alzheimer's. I had been dreading hearing this since the day Dad was diagnosed. I was also dreading the day that he would need to be placed in this unit.

If you know anything about an Alzheimer's unit of a care facility, you would understand my dread. The first characteristic of this area is that it is a locked unit. Just the connotation of putting someone that you love into a locked area is enough to break your heart. Another feature of this section is the wide range of mental deterioration that the residents have. Some are still able to converse and are very alert while some are in a zombie-like state. Dad was in the former range, so the thought of him being placed with people in the latter state was gut-wrenching to me. It was time for us to be an advocate for Dad again.

I told Randy on this phone call that there was no way that I was going to agree to this move and that Sam and I would like to have a meeting with her to discuss this in person. I wanted reasons and proof as to why she felt he should be moved to this unit. We set up a meeting for the following week.

It was time to rally the troops. I wanted Barbara to be there along with Jim, Sam, and I. I felt like there was strength in numbers. We were all going to present our case as to why Dad did not belong in the Alzheimer's unit. While we were seeing his decline, we did not feel that he was ready for that move.

For the next week, I did my research on late stage Alzheimer's disease. I wanted to dispel any thoughts that Randy had that Dad had moved to this phase of the disease. Some of the characteristics of this stage were the following: difficulty moving or walking, loss of ability to communicate through words, difficulty swallowing or eating, total incontinence of bladder and bowel, inability to hold up one's head, loss of facial expressions, including the ability to smile. There was no way that Dad was in this stage. He was still able to eat and swallow, go to the bathroom by himself (with a few accidents along the way), and converse with people. We still went for walks a few times a week, which he still loved. And he always smiled—always that beautiful, heartwarming smile. I was ready for a fight.

We showed up at our meeting with notebooks filled with examples of activities that Dad was still able to do that proved he was not in the later stages of Alzheimer's disease. I went first with my list. I told her about our long walks a few times a week, our conversations, our dinners out in which he was definitely able to swallow, and the beautiful, warm smile that he always had for me whenever I walked into the room. Sam followed with his list, then Jim, and then Barbara. They all told about the conversations that they had with Dad in which, for the most part, he was able to understand and follow. We all stated that we did not feel that he was in any way ready for this area of the facility and that he was in no way as advanced in the disease as many of the other residents were.

Randy had also done her homework and was ready for us. She had two of Dad's nurses attend our meeting. As they all listened attentively to our arguments, they took notes and nodded in agreement. But when we were finished, she hit us with a bombshell that we were not expecting. She informed us that Dad had started to wander.

I had always been concerned about this characteristic of Alzheimer's disease when Dad was living alone. I had read many articles about patients with the disease wandering and not being able to remember where they were. My brother knew of someone's parent who wandered outside to put his trash out during the winter without his coat on and then could not find his way back inside. So he roamed around outside for an hour until someone saw him and helped him back inside. I had feared this with Dad for a long time but had never seen any indication of him wandering.

Randy informed me that several of the night nurses had found Dad wandering around the halls in his underwear. On one occasion, he had gone into another resident's room and laid down on their sofa. Apparently, this roaming the halls had happened a number of times. While there was no way that he could leave the facility during the night since the main door was locked and alarmed, they were fearful that he would wander down the staircase when no one saw him and could fall and injure himself. Randy said that because of this, it was no longer possible for him to continue to stay in the assisted-living part of Briarwood.

I cried, I threatened, and I pleaded. I could not stand the thought of my father being placed in this unit. I asked her if she would agree to having Dad's doctor administer another Mini-Mental State Exam to prove that he was not in the advanced stages of Alzheimer's disease. She agreed to do this but said that that would not change her mind. For liability reasons and for his own safety, Dad would have to move.

We left the meeting feeling very defeated. I had decided that we would look for another assisted-living facility. To hell with Briarwood. I was angry that they were doing this to us, and I would not agree to this. Sam and I began looking for other facilities. In the meantime, I was waiting for the results of the MMSE so that I could prove my point.

We went to look at another facility that week. While it was nice, it was not anywhere near the caliber of Briarwood. We spoke to the director there and explained what was happening with Dad. She told us that she would need to see the results of an MMSE in order to know where to place him. She informed us that if he scored in the advanced stage of the disease, she too would have to place him in their Alzheimer's unit. I was so sure that Dad would not score in that stage that I asked her to hold a room for us in the assisted-living section.

When Sam and I left, we discussed the fact that change is very difficult for a person with Alzheimer's disease. We had seen this with Dad a great deal lately. When I would bring him to my house on a Sunday afternoon, he would constantly look at his watch and be very anxious to get "home." So did we really have his best interests at heart by moving him to another facility now, or were we just so angry with Briarwood and Randy that we were willing to sacrifice his comfort? While he would have to move to another room and another unit, he would still see the same nurses, activities coordinators, cafeteria workers, all the people that loved him and made a big fuss over him. We decided to wait for the results from the test before we made any decisions. Dad's doctor visited Briarwood once a week to check on the residents, and I had asked him to administer the test while he was visiting. He agreed to do that.

A week later, Randy called and asked Sam and I to come in to go over the results of Dad's test. We were anxious to get the results and put this to rest. So we set up a meeting with Randy for the next day.

When we got there, Randy looked upset. I thought that she was upset because we were right and Dad had scored very well. I was not ready for the shocking results.

The test is out of thirty points. Previously, Dad had scored a twenty. This time he scored an eight. Some of the answers he got incorrect were the following:

What year is this? Dad didn't know.

What season is this? Dad said spring. (It was fall.)

What month is this? Dad said April (It was September.)

What state are we in? Dad said Jersey (It was Pennsylvania.)

He was told to remember three objects because the doctor was going to ask him what they were again in a few minutes. The objects were "ball," "car," "man." When the doctor asked him a few minutes later, Dad could not remember even one of the objects.

He was asked to write a complete sentence as he had been asked on his first MMSE, and he was not able to do it.

He was given three instructions: "Take this piece of paper in your right hand, fold the paper in half, and put the paper down on the floor." Dad could not follow the instructions.

The torture went on and on. At the bottom of the test was the score 8/30. And on the next page was the diagnosis: moderately severe Alzheimer's disease. And the care recommended: most often in complex care facility. Translation: Alzheimer's unit.

I was devastated. I felt like someone had punched me in the stomach. I wanted to vomit. I wanted to scream. I wanted to punch someone. Anything but put my father in a locked Alzheimer's unit.

As I sat in Randy's office, she hugged me and told me that putting Dad in this unit would be the best place for his safety. While I realized this now in my head, my heart was broken. How was I going to do this to my father? How was I going to explain this to him? Would he even understand?

Sam and I walked out into the parking lot and cried. We knew what we had to do. We just did not know how we were going to do it and get through it. I cried the whole way home, knowing that there was no alternative. And feeling like I had the weight of the world on my shoulders as I held my father's fate in my hands.

In the next few days, we started to get ready for Dad's move. I asked Randy to please give him a room that looked exactly like his so that maybe he would not notice the move. She gave him the room directly above his present room so it looked out on the same view. She also said that she would have maintenance move his furniture and put everything in the exact same spot. They even hung the pictures on the walls in the same positions as his present room. If you did not know any better, you would think it was the same room. Unfortunately, it was not the same type of people.

This part is going to sound very pretentious of me. But my father was nothing like the people in this unit. Some of them sat and rocked back and forth all day long. Some could no longer communicate. Some slept all day. While I know he was wandering and having trouble in many areas, it did not feel to any of us that he was as disabled or that his disease was as advanced as many of the people that were there. It was so hard to see this whenever we visited.

We tried to take Dad out as much as possible. Anything to get him out of there. He seemed so sad, which made me extremely upset. I made sure he still got his newspaper every day, but he no longer read it. We all still visited regularly, so he had visitors every day. But each of us noticed that he did not fit in in this place. One day, Carla called me, crying.

She said, "Maryanne, my Sammy Sam doesn't belong there. He's nothing like the other residents there. He looks so sad."

We both cried on the phone as we realized that this was not a good fit for Dad.

I thought about quitting my job and taking him to live at my house. I discussed this with his doctor and with some of the social workers at Briarwood. They informed me of what was to come. His doctor asked me if I was prepared to change my father's diaper. Would I be able to handle that? And, most importantly, would my father? He was such a proud man. He would be horrified if he knew that I had to do that for him. And so would I.

I remember as a young girl hearing about my aunt having to bathe my elderly grandfather after he had severely broken his leg, and my grandmother was too weak to help him. My aunt relayed the story, with tears streaming down her face, about how humiliated my grandfather was at the fact that his daughter was bathing him. She said they both cried. She said there are some things a daughter should not have to do for her father. This memory came back to me when my dad's doctor asked me that question.

The doctor also asked me if I would be able to watch him around the clock. The fact that Dad was wandering would mean that I would have to alarm his bed and be ready to get to him before he could wander out the door. This was a significant safety concern that I was not sure I was able to handle.

And finally, he told me about what was to come in terms of Dad being able to eat. As I had learned previously, in the final stages of Alzheimer's disease, the patient can longer swallow. I could never understand this when I read this in much of the research that I had done on Alzheimer's. I thought that swallowing was an innate reflex, and I did not understand how that could be affected by this disease. However, the doctor explained to me that the brain no longer remembers how to swallow. At this point, the patient is either put on a feeding tube or food is withheld, and they are put on palliative care to make them comfortable as they slowly drift away. He asked me if I was prepared for this stage and if I thought I could manage this at home.

He felt that Dad's disease progression up until now had been a slow one and that we had been fortunate. But he felt that now it was "picking up speed" and that he was going to progress much more quickly at this point. Because he was now in the final stages of the disease, he felt that the incontinence, the inability to swallow and communicate, and the wandering were going to get much worse very quickly and that, for that reason, he needed to be in a constant care facility. He told me to take some time and try to think about this with my head and not my heart.

I struggled with this decision. I did not want Dad to have to live another day in the Alzheimer's unit, but I wasn't sure that I could care for him at home, especially with his progression getting worse by the day. This fact made me feel so upset with myself. What was I lacking as a person that I could not care for my father in my home?

Then I remembered another conversation from when I was a young girl. My maternal grandmother was in a nursing home, and the guilt that my mother had for putting her mother there was eating her alive. She spoke to my grandmother's doctor about taking her to live at my mom and dad's house. The doctor told my mother that this was a huge undertaking and that my mother, because of her heart condition, could, quite possibly, die before my grandmother due to the enormous stress. He felt it was in my mother's best interest to have my grandmother in a facility that could give her twenty-four-hour care.

At this point in Dad's disease, my health was starting to be affected in a significant way, so I was not sure if I could manage this responsibility physically or mentally. With unbelievable pain in my heart, I abandoned the idea of taking him home with me. The decision soon proved to be a very good one.

CHAPTER 35

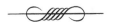

The Slippery Slope

While the progression of Dad's disease had moved relatively slowly from the time he was diagnosed in the fall of 2005 until he was moved to the Alzheimer's unit in the fall of 2013, the four months prior to his death proved to be a slippery slope of decline. Many of the final symptoms of the disease were now in full bloom. We assumed that this was what Randy had expected when she told us that he needed to be moved to continual care.

Dad had moved into the Alzheimer's unit in September. By October, his incontinence had gotten to the point that he was losing control regularly. I fought and cried about them putting a diaper on him. I begged them not to have him lose his dignity like that. However, they assured me that he no longer knew that he was wearing a diaper and that it was harder on me to see than on him. They explained that I needed to come to terms with it and realize that it was the circle of life and what he needed at this time. I finally came to accept it although seeing this proud, strong man in a diaper took a piece of my heart. This had been one of my worst fears, and it was now coming true.

Jimmy had gone to visit his grandfather one day and had decided to take him for a walk at his favorite park. Dad was still able to walk pretty well with his walker at this point, so they headed out for a loop around the walking path. As they got to the other side of the loop, Dad passed gas. Well, at least, that is what Jimmy had thought. It soon became obvious to Jimmy that Dad had lost bowel control. However, he did not want to embarrass his grandfather, so he ignored it. They continued their walk and got back to the car.

When they got into the car, Dad did not seem to realize that he had an accident, but my poor son had to deal with the odor for the entire ride back to Briarwood. He opened the windows and pretended not to notice to save Dad any embarrassment. By the time they got back to the facility, Jimmy was wrestling with how to handle the situation. He helped Dad out of the car and then motioned for a nurse standing nearby to come over. Quietly, he told the nurse what had happened, and she quickly whisked Dad away to change him.

Jimmy came home that day very upset. It was very difficult for him to see his grandfather like this. While I told him that he handled the situation beautifully, he struggled with the idea of taking Dad out for more of these outings. I agreed with him. It was getting to the point that it may be safer to just visit with him at Briarwood in the event that he had more of these accidents. This broke Jimmy's heart as he enjoyed these special times with his grandfather.

The incontinence was not the only thing that we noticed in Dad's disease progression. On one of our outings, I noticed that he was unusually quiet. His conversations had been getting progressively shorter in the past few months, but on this particular day, he was barely speaking. When I asked him if there was anything wrong, his response was heartbreaking.

He said, "Sometimes I know what I want to say here"—pointing to his head—"but I can't get it to come out right here," he added, pointing to his mouth.

I tried to make him feel better by telling him the same thing happens to me sometimes, but it broke my heart to know that he was struggling so much to speak.

At this point, Dad could no longer bathe or dress himself. An aide would bathe him a few times a week, and someone would have to dress him in the morning. If he did try to do it himself, the buttons were never done properly, and he could not figure out how to zip up his pants. This became very evident one day when I arrived to take him out for a bit. I did not realize that his pants were not zipped or buttoned. He was starting to lose weight at this point, so his pants were rather loose to begin with and not having them fastened created more of a problem. As we stepped off the elevator and Dad began walking, his pants fell down to his ankles. I was horrified. There were many people sitting around in the lobby, and I could not imagine the humiliation that this proud man must be feeling. I quickly bent down and pulled his pants back up and fastened them for him. However, to my amazement, he did not even realize what had happened. Again, there are blessings in Alzheimer's disease.

There were times that Dad was able to put on the shirts that I had bought for him without buttons, but he even needed help with that. Prior to him moving to the Alzheimer's unit, I had purchased sneakers with Velcro on them when I noticed that he was having trouble tying his sneakers. However, at this point in his decline, he could not figure out how to fasten the Velcro either. Along with the bathing and dressing, Dad was also starting to have trouble eating.

On the few occasions that I did take Dad out for dinner or just to get a quick bite to eat, I noticed that he seemed to be struggling. He would chew his food continuously, and it seemed like he was having a very difficult time with it. I took him to his dentist to see if it was his dentures. Could it be that they were not fitting properly? The dentist noticed that he had lost some weight and said that his dentures were not as snug as they used to be. So we decided to have new ones made.

The dentist took an impression of Dad's mouth, and we started the long process of having new dentures made and fitted properly so that he would be able to chew comfortably. While we were waiting for the finished product, Dad had a lot of soft foods and milkshakes. However, I noticed that he seemed to be struggling with them as well. I could not wait for the dentures to be finished so that he could eat normally again.

In December, Briarwood had their annual Christmas party. Sam, Jim, the kids, and myself were all there to celebrate with Dad. He had just gotten his new dentures, and they were fitted perfectly to his mouth, so I was so delighted that he would now be able to chew easily. We all piled our plates high with the delicious food that was being served. I got Dad's plate for him with all the things that I knew he loved. As we all sat eating, I watched Dad chew and chew. And chew. He also kept adding more food to his mouth. Finally, I noticed that the left side of his face looked like a chipmunk storing nuts.

I said, "Dad, don't put any more food in your mouth until you swallow what's there."

He looked at me blankly and did not seem to understand what I was saying. I gave him a napkin so that he could take the chewed-up food out of his mouth to speak.

He said, "Sometimes I just can't…" And with his hand going up and down his throat, he motioned that he could not swallow. He didn't even know the word for it, let alone how to do it. I felt a feeling of dread wash over me as realization started to creep in.

For months, we had thought that it was his dentures that were preventing him from eating. In reality, he was beginning to forget how to swallow. This is exactly what his doctor had told me would happen.

I quickly got up from the table to go find a nurse. I explained to her what Dad had "told" me, and she nodded. She said that they had also been noticing that he was "pocketing" his food lately and thought that perhaps we should try pureeing his food. I did not understand how this would help if he couldn't swallow, but I agreed to try anything to help him eat.

They started serving Dad's food pureed. It was a horrible sight to see. When I arrived one evening at dinner time, I sat with him and watched while the aide placed a plate in front of him with a mound of something orange and whipped. I thought it was mashed sweet potatoes. When I asked the aide what it was, she told me it was spaghetti with sauce. My poor Italian father who had grown up on homemade spaghetti and gravy, as we called it, was getting ready to eat pureed spaghetti that was served in a glob on his plate. I wanted to cry.

But perhaps even more upsetting than the wad of spaghetti that he was about to eat was the fact that he could not feed himself. When he tried to pick it up with his spoon, he did not know what to do with it. He could not figure out how to get it to his mouth. I struggled between wanting to help him but not wanting to take away his dignity. In the end, I picked up the food and began to feed my father. Life had truly come full circle.

All during the month of December, Dad's decline progressed very quickly. He was now fully incontinent, was sometimes not able to swallow, was not able to feed himself, and was conversing less and less. He was no longer interested in watching TV or reading the paper. He slept more and more of the time. He did not seem to understand when we spoke to him. And he smiled less and less, which was so sad to see, as he had always been such a happy person with a ready smile for anyone he came in contact with. I looked up the symptoms for the final stages of Alzheimer's disease, and Dad had every one of them.

His doctor spoke to me about putting Dad on hospice as he felt that he was nearing the end. Hearing the word "hospice" sounded so final to me. However, he explained that hospice would focus on keeping him comfortable and on his quality of life. It would also help all of us to prepare for his death. He was right. It was a godsend.

Hospice provided us with a counselor to speak with, and the nurses were in constant contact with us. They were able to tell us at each step of Dad's decline what to expect next. The support that they provided to us was invaluable.

The four months that Dad had been in the Alzheimer's unit had truly been a slippery slope of decline. His disease had progressed slowly over the previous eight years. However, from that initial phone call from Randy in September until the end of 2013, the progression moved with lightning speed. As much as I had fought the move, I now saw what Randy had seen and understood why she felt he needed the extra care. Sometimes it's so hard to listen to the professionals who deal with this every day. Especially when your heart is involved.

CHAPTER 36

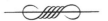

The Gifts

In the last few weeks of Dad's life, we were given many gifts. And many signs. If I had ever had any doubts about an afterlife and seeing people who had gone before me, those doubts were snuffed out while watching my father slowly leave this world. He showed all of us that there is truth to the end of life experiences that have been talked about by many people and that there have been many books written about.

The last month of Dad's life was very grueling. He was now on hospice and needed constant care. The day that I had to sign the hospice papers was one of the hardest in my life. I remember reading each paragraph, and when I got to the one about agreeing to withhold food and water from him in the final stages, I almost passed out. The hospice nurse explained to me that when people are near death, their organs start to shut down, and there is no longer a need for food. She said that I would actually be doing him more harm if I wanted them to administer a feeding tube because his body would no longer be able to process the nourishment. I was devastated. How could I sign a paper basically agreeing to starve my father? But then I remembered a conversation that Dad and I had had when he appointed me as his power of attorney, and he signed a living will years ago. He said that if he had to be kept alive artificially, then that was not really living, so he did not want any heroic measures. He wanted to be able to die peacefully. I was so thankful that we had prepared these documents before his health had declined and that we had had that conversation. That helped me to sign the hospice papers, knowing that I was carrying out Dad's wishes.

I would recommend to anyone who is caring for a loved one with Alzheimer's disease to talk to them about their last wishes. While it may be a very difficult question to ask, it will be very beneficial to you, as the caregiver, to know that you are doing what your loved one wanted at the end of their life. Also, it is very important to have this conversation at the early stages of this disease while the person is still able to understand and is of sound mind.

Not only is it important to establish your loved one's last wishes, but it is also crucial to have your loved one appoint someone as their power of attorney. This is a written authorization to represent or act on another's behalf if that person is physically or mentally incapable of managing their affairs. There are different forms of power of attorney from general power of attorney, which allows the appointed person to make financial and business transactions, to a health-care power of attorney, which grants the appointed person the ability to make medical decisions for the patient if they are unconscious, mentally incompetent, or otherwise unable to make decisions on their own. Again, this is something that is very important to do at the early stages of the disease so that your loved one understands what they are entrusting you with.

At the time that Dad was put on hospice, he was still able to eat occasionally. But other times, he was forgetting how to swallow. All his food had to be pureed, and he needed to be fed. He could no longer handle using a spoon or even figure out how to get it to his mouth. He no longer recognized certain people and could not recall names. He had lost a significant amount of weight and looked very drawn and emaciated. But perhaps the most awful of the changes that happened during this last month was the realization of one of the fears that I had had since the day Dad was diagnosed. My father did not know who I was.

I arrived one day to find Dad sleeping. I gently shook him awake to let him know that I was there. I looked forward to seeing that beautiful, huge smile on his face that he always greeted me with whenever he saw me. He slowly opened his eyes. And he looked right through me. He had no idea who I was. I spoke to him and hugged and kissed him. But he still did not know me. Another piece of my heart was ripped from my chest. How could this man who thought the sun rose and set on me and who had always called me his baby doll not know me? And then I remembered what his doctor had told me years ago at that terrible office visit about the end stages of Alzheimer's disease. This horrible disease had taken every part of my father from me. Luckily, the next day when I came to visit, I was greeted by that huge smile and a hug, and he knew, once again, that I was his daughter.

Sam and I were visiting with Dad as often as we could at this point. We knew the end was coming and wanted him to know that he was not alone. Jimmy was away at school, so he could not get there much. Katelyn went with me every time we visited him. He knew who she was, but he couldn't remember her name. One day, she asked him if he knew her name, and he said he did, but he could not tell her what it was. He called her Caesar. We had to keep from laughing in front of him.

On January 1, 2014, we went to celebrate New Year's Day with Dad. We took him out for a short walk, which he loved, and we took many pictures with him. He still had that radiant smile on his face. We stopped for Frosties, which was his special treat with Katelyn. When we fed it to him, it came right back out of his mouth. He could not remember what to do with it. We tried to show him how to swallow, but he was not able to do it. The same thing happened when we tried to give him a drink of water. It was truly heartbreaking.

Over the next few weeks, some truly awe-inspiring occurrences happened as Dad was nearing the end of his life. I learned from talking to the hospice nurse that these are called near-death experiences, and they were sincerely remarkable to witness. One day, I was sitting in his room, and he looked out the window and said, "Oh look, there's Rusty." Rusty was our dog when we were growing up, and he was Dad's little sidekick. He had died about twenty years ago.

I said, "Where is Rusty, Dad?"

And he replied, "He's out there romping around in the snow."

Another day, he looked into the distance and said, "Oh look, there's your mom."

I looked over in amazement and said, "Where, Dad?"

He pointed to the corner of the room and said, with a magnificent smile on his face, "She's standing right over there."

It made me want to cry and smile at the same time, thinking that he was seeing Mom and that she was possibly coming to greet him when he passed.

One day, when Katelyn was with him, he told her that a woman was standing in the room. He also told her that he was tired. When she told him to take a nap, he said, "No, that's okay. I'll sleep when I'm on the train." Apparently, many people at the end of their lives talk about taking a train or plane ride. In Dad's case, it was a train!

Another phenomenon that is characteristic of end of life is the experience of seeing a waterfall or stream of some sort. One day, when I was walking down the hall with Dad back to his room, he stepped widely with his legs as if he was stepping over something. When I asked what he was doing, he said he was stepping over the stream. When we got back to his room, we turned on the TV, and he commented on the beautiful waterfall on the screen. There was a commercial on for dog food; there was not a waterfall in sight.

At the time of all these occurrences, I had no idea what Dad was experiencing. I spoke to his hospice nurse about this, and she said that she had seen this numerous times over her many years of dealing with dying patients. She suggested that I read two books on the subject, *Final Journeys* by Maggie Callahan and *Final Gifts* by Maggie Callahan and Patricia Kelley. Reading these books gave me a sense of peace and awe at what Dad was experiencing at the end of his life. I would highly recommend these books to anyone going through this phase of life with a loved one.

Along with all the other incidents that Dad was experiencing, he was also exhibiting another behavior that I had read about in the books recommended by hospice. The books stated that a dying patient will reach for something that others cannot see. Dad spent many days toward the end of his life reaching to the sky. He would look up with a smile on his face and reach as if to grab at something or someone. I would ask him what he was seeing, but he never replied. He just reached and smiled a beautiful, peaceful smile.

As the days went on, I was on the phone with hospice constantly. They told me that Dad's body was starting to shut down. While I could not stand to see my father like this anymore and I had prayed that God would take him and not let him suffer anymore, the thought of losing my father was devastating. One of the hospice nurses told me that I should have a conversation with him to let him know that I was going to be okay. She said that many times people will hang on if they think that their loved ones will not be able to handle their death. She told me to tell him that it was time for him to let go.

How was I going to have this conversation with my father? The thought of it broke my heart. But it also broke my heart to see him like this. So one night, while I was visiting him, I decided to have a heart-to-heart talk with him. He looked so tired and drawn. I sat down across from him and held his hand.

I said, "Dad, we need to talk."

He said, "Okay, what do you want to talk about?"

I replied, "You look so tired."

He replied, "Yes, I am very tired."

"Dad," I started. "Sam and I are going to miss you so much. But I think that it's time that you go to heaven to be with the rest of your family. Mom is waiting for you along with your mom and dad and brothers and sister. They all want to be with you again. We can't be selfish and keep you here. So I think that it's time that you go rest."

Dad had misunderstood me and replied, "Yes, I think it is time that I go west."

I started laughing and said, "No, Dad, heaven is north, so you need to go north."

And he broke out into a hearty laugh and said, "You're right. I think it's time I go north." Then a remarkable, mysterious occurrence happened. He looked at my right shoulder and said, "What is that on your shoulder?"

When I looked puzzled and asked him what he saw, he began tracking with his eyes to my other shoulder and then around the room with a beatific smile on his face. It was as if he was seeing something or someone in the room. The hair on the back of my neck stood up. Was there an angel in the room with us? Was Mom here to take him home? It was such a special, beautiful experience. I had given Dad permission to go home. And we were both at peace.

In the last few weeks of his life, he became very expressive and appreciative with me. While he had always appreciated everything that I had done for him, he especially showed it during this period of time. Every time that I was with him, he made sure to thank me for what I was doing for him. And after each time he thanked me, he would call me his baby doll. Growing up, I always remember Dad affectionately calling me by that nickname. So it became even more special during these last few weeks with him.

He would hug and kiss me and say, "Thank you so much, baby doll. You're such a sweetheart." It meant so much to me. But I also knew that, in his way, he was saying goodbye.

Carla was with Dad one afternoon near the end, and the story that she told us about her time with him was incredible. Apparently, Dad's life was passing before his eyes that afternoon. She said that he was talking about having to go out and work on the farm that day. He told her that he had a lot of chores to do and needed to get started. She convinced him that he could get to them later and that he should just relax for a bit. Then he began to army crawl across the floor and "dig" with an imaginary shovel. When she asked him what he was doing he said that he was digging a foxhole. Then he was "carrying something" over his shoulder, and when Carla asked him what he was doing, he said he was carrying an injured soldier to safety. Carla sat in awe as she watched this reel of Dad's life unfold before her eyes.

When Barbara was with him one day that week, she said that he was very tired, so she told him to lie down and take a nap. She covered him with a blanket and sat in the room with him while he slept. After a while, he began to mumble. She could not understand what he was saying, but then suddenly he started to laugh.

And he said, "Hey, Joe, what's it like up there?"

Barbara had no idea who Joe was. When she told me about it that evening, I told her that Joe was his brother whom he was very close to and who had died many years ago.

She said, "Well, Maryanne, he definitely saw his brother because he was talking to him in his sleep."

Not only had he seen my mother, but he had also seen his brother. It was truly astonishing to see Dad experiencing this.

Dad stopped eating the week before he died. We tried to feed him, but he no longer wanted to eat or drink. We wet his lips with wet paper towels and lemon swabs that hospice had given us. He began to sleep more and more and was not conversing with us any longer. The weekend before Dad died, Jimmy came home from college to see him. We all sat in his room and spoke to him, but he did not respond. We rubbed his arms and head and told him that we were all there with him and that we loved him. When it came time for Jimmy to leave, I said, "Dad, Jimmy has to leave to head back to college now." He had not responded or moved all day. As Jimmy leaned down to kiss his grandfather, Dad lifted his arm with the little strength that he had and tried to hug Jimmy. It was amazing to see and was Dad's last gift to Jimmy. I walked him out to his car, and we cried and hugged as he talked about what an amazing grandfather he had been and how much he was going to miss him. I always felt so bad that he had to drive back to school that day, knowing that he would not see his grandfather alive again.

The following day, Katelyn came to see Dad. She walked in with a Frosty and said, "Pappers, I brought you your favorite, a chocolate Frosty."

I said, "Oh, honey, that was so nice, but he's not eating anymore."

Dad was awake that day but very lethargic. We had propped him up in a chair, and when he saw Katelyn, he smiled. Then when she tried to feed him, he began to eat the Frosty for her! Again, an amazing gift. That was their special treat together, and it was almost as if he was saying he wanted to share that one final Frosty together.

Sam and I had been taking turns staying with Dad over the past few nights. We could tell he was nearing the end, and we did not want him to be alone. It was Sam's turn to stay, and that is when

Sam received his gift from Dad. Growing up, our father was not very expressive. He rarely said I love you, and unfortunately, he never said it to Sam. In Dad's day, men did not tell each other they loved each other. While he did not say it much to me when we were growing up, he began to say it often toward the end of his life. But, again, he never said it to Sam. On this particular night, Sam was sitting next to Dad's bed talking to him, and Dad said, "I love you, Sam." It was such a special gift that meant so much to my brother. Sam told me about it the next morning, and we both cried.

Two days before Dad died, I had been at work. Sam was with him, and the hospice nurse told him that Dad only had a few days left. He called me at work to let me know. I told my boss that I had to leave and did not know when I would be back because I needed to stay with my father. He was very understanding and told me to take whatever time I needed.

I went home to pack a bag so that I could stay with Dad over the next few days, and I headed out. However, it was snowing heavily, so I had to drive very slowly. I was on the phone with Sam as I was trying to make my way there, and he told me that Dad was not responding. I was afraid he would pass before I got there, so I told Sam to tell him that I was on my way and that I would be there as soon as I could. The drive, which normally took fifty minutes, took me over two hours.

When I got there, I ran down the hall to Dad's room and burst through the door. He was sleeping and unresponsive. I sat down on the bed next to him and said, "Dad, I'm here." And then I was given the most amazing gift that I have ever received. My father lifted both arms, put them around me and, with the little strength that he had left, kissed me repeatedly. It was truly the most beautiful moment I could have ever imagined. After that moment, he slipped into a coma and never awoke.

Over the next two days, Sam and I stayed in Dad's room with him, rubbing his arms and head, telling him that we loved him and that we were there with him. The nurses would come in to bathe him and check on him from time to time, but he never responded. At one point, Dad started to exhibit the death rattle, which is part of the dying process. It occurs when the dying person is no longer able to swallow, cough, or clear saliva or mucus from the back of the throat. I had heard of this occurrence in the past but had never seen anyone experience it. It was the most awful sound that I had ever heard. It sounded like he was drowning, and it made me very upset. The nurses assured me that although it sounded terrible, Dad was feeling no pain or discomfort. He had been put on morphine to relieve any discomfort, so I was at peace with that.

On Thursday, January 23, 2014, the hospice nurse told us that Dad would probably be gone within the next day. I had not showered in a few days and desperately needed to freshen up. So Sam stayed with Dad while I ran home to do this. While I was at home, I decided to bring my iPod and a speaker to play a song that was very special to Dad and me. I had heard that hearing was the last sense to go when a person is dying, so I wanted to dedicate this special song to him in the hopes that he would hear it and remember what it meant to us.

When I was about twelve, we were going to attend a family wedding. I wanted to be able to slow dance with my dad, uncles, and anyone else that would dance with me. I asked Dad if he would teach me. So every night after dinner, we would turn on my tape recorder and play a song that was very popular at the time. It was called, "You Make Me Feel Brand New" by the Stylistics. Dad would patiently move me around the living room while I stepped on his feet, tried to lead, and basically did everything wrong. Even though I was hopeless at slow dancing, each night, he would get the tape recorder out and turn on this beautiful song. At the time, I did not pay attention to the words. But now the words were so poignant and meaningful: "You make me feel brand new, for God blessed me with you. / Only you, believed in me through thick and thin, / How can I repay you for having faith in me." I wanted to play this for Dad and tell him how blessed I felt to have him as my father and for always believing in me.

I got back to Briarwood as quickly as I could and carried the iPod and speaker in. I had my playlist up and had it set to the song. I had the speaker off but pushed play so that it would start right in on the words when I turned the speaker on. I couldn't wait to play it for Dad. I knelt down by him and held this hand.

I said, "Dad, I want to play a song for you that is so special to me and will always remind me of you. This will always be our song, Dad."

Katelyn and Sam were in the room, and they both started to cry. It was a very emotional moment. I turned on the speaker and waited for this beautiful, moving song. As I turned it on, out blasted "I'm on the Highway Hell." I must have accidentally hit the shuffle button, and it went to another song on my playlist. Laughter broke out as we all realized that "Highway to Hell" by AC/DC is probably not an appropriate song to play for someone who is dying! If Dad were conscious, he would have had a hearty laugh at that.

Once I got the playlist back to where I wanted it, I played the song for Dad and hugged him and cried. I told him how much I loved him and how blessed I felt to have him in my life. And how much I appreciated him for always having faith in me. It was a heart-wrenching, bittersweet moment.

Later in the day, Sam decided to go outside for some fresh air and to take a break from the stress and anguish of watching Dad slowly pass away. I had also moved to the other side of the room to take a short hiatus from the heartache of watching this. At that moment, the nurses came in to check on Dad, and he took his last breath. I truly believe that he waited until we were no longer by his side because he did not want us to witness that. He was trying to protect us until the very end.

When I realized that he was gone, I raced to his side and told him again how much I loved him and to rest in peace. Sam came back in after Dad had gone, and we all hugged him and cried. When word traveled through Briarwood that Dad had passed, some of the residents and nurses who loved him came to say their goodbyes. As I stated earlier, Barbara came to say goodbye and told Dad how much he meant to her. We called the funeral director that we had planned on using, and he told us he would be there in an hour. We stayed with Dad until he came, and then with a final kiss and many tears, we left his room for the last time.

Our father was at peace—no more confusion, no more forgetting, no more not knowing how to do basic things like using the bathroom, feeding himself, and swallowing. As hard as it was to see this great man leave this earth, it was a relief to know that he was not suffering anymore. I told myself this repeatedly over the next few days as we prepared for Dad's funeral.

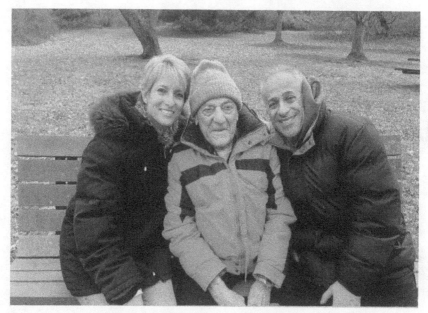

New Year's Day 2014

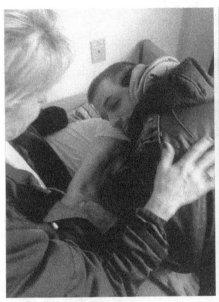 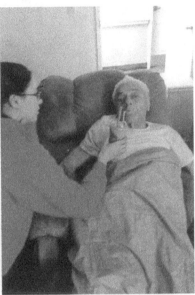

Dad hugging Jimmy goodbye with the little strength that he had left.

Eating a Frosty that Katelyn brought him. He had not eaten for days, but he attempted to eat it for her.

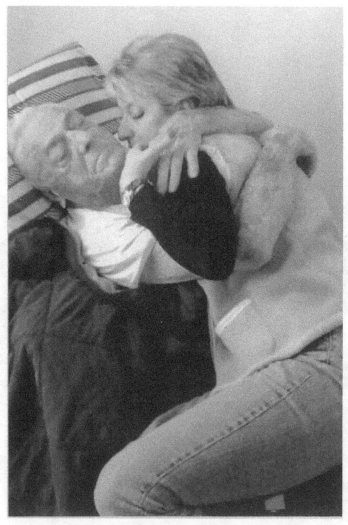

Hugging me goodbye. Dad slipped into a coma
after that and never regained consciousness

CHAPTER 37

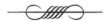

Dad's Funeral

How do you honor a man who was so honorable? Who was so kind and loving? Who loved life and his family? And who loved his country and was so proud of his service to his country? We thought about all of this as we were putting together our private funeral for Dad.

As I had said, Sam and I were exhausted from the many months of caring for Dad, and we did not have the energy to put together an elaborate service. We just wanted something private to honor this very simple, proud man. And that is what Dad would have wanted. He was not showy or pretentious, so he would not have wanted anything over the top. So we decided to honor him in a private, special way. We also wanted to honor the fact that he was a World War II veteran, so we contacted the Veterans Administration and requested military honors at his funeral.

We decided to have only myself, Sam, Jim, Jimmy, and Katelyn there. And, of course, Barbara and Carla, since they had played such a huge roll in Dad's life. Carla had just started a new job and could not take the time off, which we definitely understood. We knew that she was with him in thought. I had suggested that we write special letters to Dad that we would read to him at the funeral.

As we were preparing for the funeral, we were all coming up with things that we wanted to place in Dad's casket with him. All the things that were special to him. They included his *Reader's Digest*, a deck of playing cards, a Hershey chocolate bar, and a picture collage of all of us with him.

I had been to many funerals over the course of my life. In many cases, the deceased were dressed in a suit or dress. I had only seen Dad in a suit on a handful of occasions. That just was not his style. His typical way of dressing was in casual pants, a button-down shirt with a pocket for his glasses, and his Reebok sneakers. So that is how Sam and I decided to dress him for his final journey.

When we arrived at the funeral home, I knew that it was going to be a tough day. While I was happy that Dad was no longer suffering and confused, I also knew that I was saying a final goodbye to a man who had meant so much to me. A man who had been by my side for fifty-two years, loving me, encouraging me, and being my biggest cheerleader. How was I going to get through this?

As we walked into the room, I looked at the casket and saw Dad looking so peaceful and serene. But the most important thing that I noticed was that he did not have that look of confusion on his face anymore. He was truly at peace. And he looked like he always did—in his casual blue pants and his button-down shirt with his glasses in his pocket. And peeking out of the blanket that was over his legs was his new pair of Reebok sneakers. It made me smile.

We all gathered around Dad while the priest said a prayer and blessed him. Then one by one, we all took out our letters that we had written to him. The most amazing thing to me was that none of us had collaborated with each other, but yet we all said basically the same thing. Jimmy and Katelyn both referred to their grandfather as a "simple man" who was happy as long as he had his watch and his wallet. They both told him what a significant impact that he had on their lives. It made me so proud to hear how my children honored my father. Following are the letters written by my amazing children to their grandfather:

Dear "Pappers,"

I wanted to write this letter to you because I wanted to tell you all of the things that I may not have told you before. I wanted to start by saying thank you. Thank you for being such a big part of my life and for being the best grandfather that I could have ever asked for. From the moment I was born until the very end, I knew that you adored me. This was proven true when you got on a crazy, spinning ride with me when you were 80 years old. That is something not every grandfather would do for their grand-daughter. I wanted to let you know that I adore you too. You were an amazing person, Grandfather, and friend.

The next point I wanted to mention is something I never told you, but now I wish I had. You were one of only a select number of people who has had the biggest influence on my life. You taught me some of the most important lessons and I bet you didn't even realize it. The first lesson you taught me was to be kind to everyone. I have never met a man who was as kind-hearted as you. You truly had a heart of gold. Never once did I hear you say a mean thing about anyone, and everyone who ever crossed your path was met with a hearty smile. The people who knew you should know how lucky they were to have known such a gracious gentleman, because they will never meet anyone better.

The second and most important lesson I learned from you is to enjoy the simple things in life. I admired how humble you were. You were the definition of the "American Dream." You didn't have the easiest life, but you overcame many hardships, you fought for your country and you had a successful career. Not to mention the fact that you had a perfect family and you helped raise two wonderful children, who I know you were so extremely proud of. Grandpop, you had every reason to brag about yourself, but you didn't because that is not the kind of man you were. You were a simple man, a man who valued his $10-dollar watch and having $3 dollars in his wallet. That's all that you needed to make you happy. You didn't need anything big. For you, the littlest things meant the most. That is such an admirable trait. You found so much joy in going for walks so you could "get a whiff of this fresh air," and eating your beloved Frosties, which I will always have the honor of being the last person you ate one with. I'm going to carry out your simple lifestyle because you showed me that the simpler a person's life is, the happier they are. Seeing you get excited over little things brought me so much joy. If all people on earth were as gracious and appreciative as you were, we would live in an absolute paradise.

I could go on forever about how much you meant to me and how you impacted my life in so many ways. While I am going to miss you very much, I'm so happy for you that you are reunited with your other family and that you are no longer in pain. I take comfort in knowing that I now have a permanent Angel looking out for me. But the point I wanted to end my letter with, and the point that I definitely made sure you knew while you were here, was that I loved you so very much. How I got so lucky to have such an awesome Grandpop, I'll never know. But, I'm very blessed. I'm blessed and honored to have known such a wonderful, easy-going, kind-hearted, funny, caring man. I love you more than you will ever know, and I thank God every day that I had you as my Grandpop.

Love Always,
"Katie-Baby"

Dear Grandpop,

As I sit here writing this letter, I find myself faced with a difficult task. I am racking my brain trying to find one word that best describes you and that summarizes who you are and I realize that this is impossible because there isn't one word that describes you. There are many. Many people would agree with me that it would take forever and a day to create a comprehensive list of all of the great traits that make you who you are. However, on behalf of the many people that love you, I'd like to take the time to share with you a few of the traits that we will always remember you for and that have made you the fantastic person that you are. You are friendly to everybody you meet and never say a bad thing about anybody, you are hardworking, caring, sensitive, committed to your family and friends, optimistic, good-humored, tough, determined, and a virile fighter. It is for all of these traits that you will be forever in our hearts and we will always love you.

If I could pick the one word that describes you that has had the most lasting and significant impact on me, it would be this: simple. It never took much to make you happy because just being alive was enough for you and you looked at each day as a gift. You made it a point to love life each and every day and the way you presented yourself to the world showed this. With your plaid, buttoned-down shirt with your reading glasses in the pocket, jeans, sneakers, hat, wristwatch, and wallet you showed the world how down-to-earth you really are and that you are not wrapped up in the trivial, expensive items of today's materialistic world. It never mattered how much money was in your wallet, just as long as it was on you at all times, as it was a part of the image of a down-to-earth man that enjoyed life's simple pleasures.

I will always remember and treasure the fun times we had together. Between having a catch in the backyard, playing Bingo, watching TV, going to the Italian Market in Philadelphia, going on roller coasters at Great Adventure, going for walks at the Farm Park, getting lunch and enjoying Frosties at Wendy's, or just sitting on the beach talking and enjoying a good laugh, you were always happy because you were enjoying life with people that you loved and that loved you back. I always loved every second I spent with you and could not wait until the next time I was able to see you again. I always felt that you were more than a grandfather; you were a friend and a teacher. You taught me that the best things in life are not things, but time spent doing what you love with who you love and the memories that come from these wonderful experiences.

Words cannot even begin to express how much you mean to me and how much of an impact you have had on my life. You are one of the greatest men I've ever known and I am going to miss you terribly. Thank you so much for making the last 23 years of my life so wonderful and special. I love you so much and I will always have a special place in my heart for you.

Love,
Jimmy

Jim's letter was truly amazing. He thanked my dad for being a wonderful father-in-law and for accepting him into the family with open arms. He thanked him for me and for the many years that we all had together. He read the letter with tears in his eyes, and his voice quavering with emotion. It was such a beautiful tribute.

Sam also thanked Dad for being an amazing father and for always being there to support him. He struggled to get through it, but with tears streaming down his face, he was able to read his incredible tribute to our father.

Now it was my turn. I took my letter out of my pocket and held Dad's hand while I read it to him.

Dad,

I've been thinking over the last few weeks about all of the things that you have taught me over the years. You taught me how to ride a bike, how to slow dance, how to drive a car. You even taught me how to change a tire. But one thing you didn't teach me was how to go through the rest of my life without you. I guess I'll have to figure that out on my own.

The most important thing that I want to learn from you, though, is how to be the wonderful person that you were. The words that were used to describe you over the last week have truly inspired me: wonderful, kind, caring, one of a kind, the unique quality of making people feel special, thoughtful. The list goes on. I can only hope to aspire to be half the person you were.

The other thing I want to learn from you is how to be strong. I used to joke that you were like the Energizer Bunny because you just kept going on and on. You made it through the war, mom's death, a stroke, a heart attack, and many other trials and tribulations throughout your life. But through everything, you were always pleasant and just kept plugging along. I need to learn to be strong like you.

One more thing I want to learn from you is how to be good at everything. You were awesome at everything you did. You were a terrific son and brother. An amazing husband. A remarkable father. A wonderful father-in-law. An incredible grandfather. And a kind and caring friend. Oh, and I can't forget a brave soldier. There wasn't anything that you didn't do perfectly. I'll have to strive for that perfection also.

I hope you know how much I truly loved you. I know I seemed impatient with you at times, but I think I was just always so angry at this horrible disease and how it robbed me of the dad I used to know. I hated seeing you so confused and lost. But knowing that you are at peace now and happy with mom and your other family makes me feel so much better.

You will always be in my heart. You will always be an inspiration to me. You will always be my Energizer Bunny. And I will always be your baby doll.

I love you Dad.

Your daughter forever,
Maryanne

As I finished reading my letter to Dad, I bent down and kissed him. I placed my letter in his pocket and took his glasses out so that I could keep them to remember him by. The kids, Jim, and Sam tucked their letters in with Dad. Since I had always referred to Dad as the Energizer Bunny, I spent the days before his funeral trying to find a stuffed Energizer Bunny to place in the casket, but I was not able to find one. So instead, I found a white teddy bear holding a heart that said, "I Love You." I placed that next to Dad's head. Then we pulled his blanket up and all gave him a final kiss as we cried and hugged each other.

We followed the hearse to Saint Patrick's cemetery and to Dad's final resting place. Before being brought to the grave, the casket was brought to the cemetery chapel. As we pulled up, two uniformed Army officers stood at attention. As Dad's flag-draped casket was taken out of the hearse, the officers saluted him. Then we all went into the chapel for Dad's military send off.

The priest said a few prayers over Dad's casket and blessed him. Then the officers lifted the flag and held it taut over the casket. At that moment, from the back of the chapel, a bugler began playing "Taps." We all held each other and cried at this poignant, beautiful moment. As the bugler finished playing, the officers began folding the flag into a perfect triangle. When they finished, one of the officers came over and presented the flag to Sam. As he handed him the flag, he said, "On behalf of the president of the United States, the United States Army, and a grateful nation, please accept this flag as a symbol of our appreciation for your loved one's honorable and faithful service." Then he saluted him. While it was a very sad moment for all of us, it was also a moment filled with immense pride in this honorable soldier.

As we walked out into the dreary January day, we thanked the officers for the beautiful tribute to our father. We all followed the hearse to the gravesite and our final goodbye.

As we pulled up to the open grave, I remember wishing that it had been a sunny day, which was Dad's favorite kind, instead of the gloomy, cloudy day that it was. We got out of the cars and waited as the funeral director opened the back of the hearse. As he began to pull Dad's casket out to place it on the bier, we all gasped. The clouds parted, and the sun began to shine. We all looked at each other and smiled. The sun had come out especially for Dad.

As we walked behind the bier to his grave, we were each given a carnation by the funeral director. The priest said a final prayer, and we all placed our flowers on the casket. I looked at the tombstone that had Mom's name on it and smiled as I realized that my parents were together again after almost thirty years apart. I was going to miss my father so much. But I was so happy that he and Mom were together and that he was resting in peace.

As we got into our cars to drive away, I gave one final look back at the casket that held the man who had meant so much to me. And I smiled through my tears. It was a beautiful send off for a wonderful father, grandfather, father-in-law, son, friend, and brave soldier.

CHAPTER 38

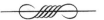

Now What Do I Do?

In the weeks after Dad's death, I felt a profound sense of loss. While I was so relieved that he was no longer suffering the confusion and debilitation of Alzheimer's disease, I missed him tremendously. I missed his smile. I missed his presence. And I missed having the man who was by my side since day one, protecting me and guiding me through life. I felt so incredibly despondent and brokenhearted. I also felt lost and adrift.

One of the hardest adjustments after someone with a long illness, that you have been caring for, dies is what to do with yourself. You've been a caregiver for such a long time that you do not know what else to do with that time. Your whole life has been wrapped around the person who has needed you through their illness. So while you are grieving over the loss of your loved one, you are also feeling an emptiness and lack of purpose.

After Dad's death, I found myself trying to figure out what my purpose was now. I was still a wife, mother, and Educational Assistant. But my children were independent at this point and did not need me as much. I felt that I had been a caregiver for so long that I needed someone else to help. Along came another angel sent from above.

In my role as an Educational Assistant, I provided support for six sixth-grade teachers. This support came in the form of providing help in math, social studies, and science classes and pulling students out of class who were struggling in these areas to work with them one on one if the teacher felt that they needed it. It was very rewarding to be able to help these students to achieve their goals.

One day in February 2014, about three weeks after Dad had died, I walked into a sixth-grade math classroom at the start of class. As I walked in, the teacher came toward me with a look of concern on her face. She motioned for me to follow her out into the hallway. I anxiously followed her, wondering what it was that was causing her to look so upset.

When we were out of earshot of her classroom full of students, she said, "Maryanne, I need your help. A new student just joined our class who moved here from Ethiopia. He was adopted from an orphanage there by one of the families in our school, and he has never been to school before. I cannot have this child sit in my math class every day while we're learning Algebra. He will be so lost."

I looked at her disbelievingly. I knew what she wanted me to do. I knew that she wanted me to take him out of class every day and work with him, but where did I start? If he had never been to school, what was he capable of doing? Could he add, subtract, multiply? The teacher did not know what his abilities were. I was about to find out.

She went into her classroom and brought out the new student. And I was instantly captivated. As the teacher introduced him to me, he put his hand out to shake mine and told me it was a pleasure to meet me. As I looked into his huge, trusting eyes, I knew that I had found my purpose.

The child's name was Abraham, and he was thirteen years old. He had grown up on the streets in Ethiopia when he was young, having been abandoned by his mother. When he was brought to the orphanage at nine years old, he finally had a home, but the education there was very minimal. I discovered in the first few days of working with him that the only concept in math that he knew how to do was addition. I knew we had a long road ahead of us.

Each day, I went to Abraham's classroom and brought him with me to my classroom for an hour and a half. Once I felt that he had mastered addition, we moved on to subtraction. He was a whiz. He picked it up immediately. Next, I made a packet of multiplication flash cards with facts from one to ten for him to study and told him that he had to memorize all his multiplication facts. I told him to take his time and let me know when he was ready for me to test him. A week later, he came in with the pack of cards and told me he had memorized them all! He was an incredible student.

In the next few months of school, Abraham and I worked on multiplication, division, fractions, telling time, money, and geometry. And each day that he left my room, he would thank me for helping him to learn. In all the years that I had worked as an Educational Assistant, I had never worked with a student who was so eager to learn and who valued education as much as he did. And who was so appreciative of the help he was given. It was truly a wonderful experience for me.

Over the course of our months together, Abraham also told me heartbreaking stories of his time in Ethiopia. Stories about growing up on the streets, about never owning a pair of shoes, and of living in a trash dump and scrounging for food. However, as he told me these stories, there was never a moment of self-pity. He would just relay them to me in a nonchalant way that left me in shock. Many days, I would suppress my tears while we were together, only to break down sobbing after he left my room. How could this boy who had lived such a terrible life, be so kind, so appreciative, and so full of life? He was an amazing young man.

One day, Abraham came into my classroom and asked me to teach him something other than math. I said, "Of course, Abraham. What would you like to learn?" His reply left me in tears. He said, "I would like to learn the Pledge of Allegiance because now I live in America, and I love America." We proceeded to recite it over and over until he could say it himself. And, of course, he said it proudly with his hand over his heart.

Every night, I would print out worksheets for him to work on the next day. He loved homework and constantly asked me for assignments and math sheets to complete. It was my focus every day to bring Abraham one step closer to where he needed to be before he headed off to seventh grade and middle school the next year.

At the end of the school year, Abraham's mother sent me a beautiful card, thanking me for my work with him. She also asked me to meet her for coffee so that she could meet me in person. When we did, she told me that her family considered me an angel and that they were so grateful for all that I had done for their son.

With tears in my eyes, I explained what her son had done for me. I told her about my father and how I had cared for him through the many years of his decline and how lost I felt when he had gone. And how, a few weeks after his death, when I was feeling so lost and without purpose in my life, along came this gift from God. This child that gave me a reason to get up each morning with a goal in mind and a smile on my face. This child who helped me answer the question, "Now what do I do?"

I will always be grateful that Abraham came into my life when he did. We still keep in touch, and I see him from time to time at my church. He always has a ready smile for me and a big hug. And now that he has graduated high school and is heading off to college, I have an immense sense of pride at all that he has accomplished. And an immense sense of gratitude to this amazing young man for filling a huge void in my life.

CHAPTER 39

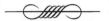

Signs

I do not know how other people feel about the idea of signs from loved ones from the afterlife, but I was a skeptic before Dad died. I had heard others talk about getting a "sign" from their deceased mother or brother or uncle. But I had never experienced that even though I had lost a lot of family members in my life. When my mother died, I looked for messages from her letting me know that she was okay, that she was still with me. But I never saw or felt anything.

I have heard it said that you have to be open to the signs, that you have to believe. Maybe I was just too angry and felt cheated after my mom's death to be "open" to any signals that may have been there. Or maybe I was just too much of a skeptic and did not really believe in signs from the afterlife.

I cannot say that I was much of a believer in near-death experiences before the encounters with my dad either. Again, I had heard about people who were dying and saw angels and loved ones who had died before them. However, I had never experienced it, so I was a skeptic. Then my dying father started seeing his deceased wife, talking to his deceased brother, and reaching for unseen objects while smiling a beautiful, peaceful smile. It made a believer out of me.

When Dad died, I wanted desperately to know that he was at peace, that he was not suffering anymore. I looked for messages or signs everywhere from him. However, I could not find any. And, as

I stated, I was not sure if I really believed in them. Until the garage door happened.

We have a two-car attached garage at our house. However, we do not use it for our cars. Like many people, we use if for storage and junk. And we pass through it on our way from the house to where our cars are parked in the driveway. We always use the left side of the garage on our route to our cars.

About three months after Dad's death, I was feeling so low and lost without him. I felt so desperate to know that he was finally at peace after all the years of confusion and disorientation. I could not seem to find the peace that I needed to move on with my life.

One beautiful, sunny day in April, I was leaving for work in the morning. I pushed the button on the wall to open the left-side garage door to get out to my car. I said goodbye to Jim and walked out into the garage. As I was walking to the door, I saw Dad's rollator walker in the corner. I went over to it, rubbed the handle, and said, "Oh, Dad, I just wish I knew if you were okay." Then I continued on to my car, which was parked in the driveway next to Jim's car.

As I reached to open my car door, I noticed that the right-side garage door began to open. I climbed into my car and realized that Jim must have opened the garage door and must be going out also. So I sat in my car and waited for him to come out. I wondered why he was opening the door on the right side of the garage since we never used that. After waiting a few minutes and realizing that he was not coming out, I called him on his cell phone.

When he answered the phone, I asked, "Are you leaving the house now, hon?"

He responded, "No, I'm watching TV."

I said, "Well, why did you open the garage door?"

And he replied, "I didn't open the garage door. I've been sitting here since you left."

I sat in bewilderment as I tried to find an explanation for how the door had opened if neither Jim nor I had hit the button to open it. Was there a mechanical malfunction? An electrical surge? Or was there another explanation for it? A strange feeling came over me. Could it possibly have been a sign from my father?

When I told Jim what I had said to my dad and what had happened, he said, "Maybe your dad was letting you know that he's okay."

Could that have been it? Was it possible for deceased loved ones to send you signs like this?

Again, I turned to books. I went to the library to see if there were books on signs from the afterlife and found an entire section dedicated to the topic. One of the first books I read was *Hello from Heaven* by Bill and Judy Guggenheim. The authors conducted a research project on after-death communications or ADCs. These are spiritual experiences that occur when you are contacted spontaneously by a deceased family member or friend without the use of psychics or mediums. It is estimated that 20 to 40 percent of the population of the United States have had one or more ADC experiences.

The Guggenheim's ADC project started in 1988 and went on for seven years. Together, they interviewed 2,000 people and collected more than 3,300 firsthand accounts of ADCs from people from all walks of life and diverse social, economic, and educational backgrounds. According to the Guggenheim's research, there are twelve frequent types of ADCs that people report having with their deceased loved ones. They are the following: sensing a presence, hearing a voice, feeling a touch, smelling a fragrance, visual experiences, visions, twilight experiences, ADCs during sleep, out-of-body ADCs, telephone calls, physical phenomenon (lights blinking on and off and mechanical objects being turned on or operated), and symbolic signs (rainbows, butterflies, coins, etc.). As I was reading this book, I zeroed in on the physical phenomenon ADC.

The Guggenheim's research concluded that many people have an ADC involving unusual physical or "poltergeist" occurrences following the death of a relative or friend that the Guggenheim's call "ADCs of physical phenomena." Examples include lights being turned on and off; radios, stereos, televisions, and other electrical devices being turned on; mechanical objects being activated; and pictures and other items being moved.

According to other books that I read on ADCs, it is common for spirits to communicate through electricity by manipulating many of these objects. I read story after story of people experiencing electrical objects being turned off and on with no explanation as to how this was done. In some cases, it was lights. In other cases, it was a radio or television. For others, it was not an electrical item but an object being moved to a different location than it was previously in. In each of these scenarios, there was no logical explanation for how these occurrences happened.

Over the many years since the opening of the garage door, I have not told many people for fear that they would think I had gone over the deep end. While the books that I read reassured me that other people had also experienced strange circumstances after the death of a loved one, I still was not quite sure if it was something I felt comfortable talking about. Did I want to include this story in my book?

One evening, as I was writing this chapter, I asked Jim if he thought that readers of my book would think I was unbalanced for writing about this topic. Was it crazy to think that our deceased loved ones send us signs and messages? He stated that some people do believe in ADCs and that, since this was something that happened after Dad's death, I should include it. I proceeded to write this chapter while still not quite sure if I wanted to include it.

Later that evening, while I was writing, Jim was in the laundry room putting a load of clothes in the washing machine when I heard him say, "What the heck is going on?"

I went in to investigate what was making him frustrated and noticed that the laundry room light kept flickering off and on. We chalked it up to the fact that the bulb must be going dead and vowed to change it the next day. We forgot about it over the next few days as we went in and out of the laundry room, turning the light on each time. Then I realized that the light was no longer flickering. The bulb was fine. And Jim and I were no longer talking about whether we believed in after-death communications. Coincidence? I don't know.

While I still have some doubts about ADCs and signs from the afterlife, all I know is there was no logical explanation for our garage door opening on its own that day that I needed so desperately to know that my father was okay. There was no electrical failure, no power surge, and neither Jim nor I had opened it. So I would like to believe that my father was sending me a sign, telling me that he was at peace and no longer suffering confusion and bewilderment. And I am sure that if he was sending me a sign, he was having a hearty laugh at my own confusion and bewilderment as to how the garage door opened!

CHAPTER 40

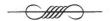

Getting Involved

Along with my new sense of purpose in working with Abraham, I also found myself reading many books on near-death experiences in the months after Dad died. I had experienced death many times in my life with my mother's passing, along with three grandparents and many aunts and uncles. But I had never seen some of the phenomena that Dad had exhibited. So I set out to educate myself on what I had seen.

I found myself smiling and nodding through many of the books that I read. Dad had experienced many of the things that I was reading. He had seen waterfalls and streams, he talked about taking a train ride, and he had seen his life passing before him. But one of the main themes in every book I read about NDEs, and that Dad had clearly experienced, was the presence of loved ones that had gone before him.

When a loved one is dying, you have a fear of where they are going and what will happen to them. I know that many people do not believe in heaven or an afterlife. As I said, over the course of my life, I have had my own doubts. But having experienced what I did with Dad has put those doubts to rest.

When Barbara called me to tell me about Dad asking my Uncle Joe what it was "like up there," I truly believed he was seeing his loved ones who had gone on to the hereafter. He and his brother Joe were very close and knowing that he had seen him, gave me a sense of peace.

When Dad had seen "something" on my shoulder the night I spoke to him about going to rest, and he had tracked that something around the room, I knew that he was truly experiencing something magical. When he saw my mother and got that huge smile on his face, I felt elated to know that Mom was there for him. And when he saw his little sidekick, Rusty, "romping around in the snow," I remember thinking that our pets must go on to the hereafter also. All these experiences gave me a sense of peace in knowing that Dad was not alone on his journey to the afterlife.

Reading these books and comparing what I read with what we experienced with Dad was a huge help in the healing process for me. I would highly recommend this practice to anyone who has any doubts about where their loved ones go when they leave this world.

Another experience that helped me in the healing process was getting involved in a cause. I hated Alzheimer's disease. I wanted to know how I could help to alleviate the pain and fear that this horrible disease causes. So I reached out to the Alzheimer's Association.

They told me about something called the Walk to End Alzheimer's. It is the world's largest event to raise awareness and funds for Alzheimer's care, support, and research. It is held annually in more than six hundred communities nationwide. There was going to be one near us in Philadelphia in November of 2014. I was definitely interested.

I registered all five of us and came up with a name for our little group. We were going to be called "Papper's Pals," and we were going to start fundraising to be able to contribute to this great cause. I put out a letter at work, explaining what we were doing and why, and many people contributed. Sam also raised money where he worked, and we made donations in Dad's memory.

We all showed up at Citizens Bank Park on the day of the Alzheimer's walk, wearing our purple Alzheimer's T-shirts. Sam brought Sadie and Ava, and we put purple bandanas around their necks so that they could be part of the festivities also. Spinning Promise Flowers were handed out to represent what each person was walking for. Purple signified that you lost someone to Alzheimer's, yellow meant you were caring for someone with the disease, blue meant that you had the disease, and orange symbolized that you supported the cause.

Participants gathered for a beautiful opening ceremony at the start of the walk in which they announced how much money was raised for the event. Then everyone raised their Promise Flower, and there was a tremendous, dynamic sea of color that created a "garden" as everyone began to walk for this rewarding fundraiser.

This is a very worthwhile cause and a wonderful community event to get involved in. I would highly recommend this for anyone who has experienced the sorrow of Alzheimer's disease. It gives you a sense of purpose and helps you to feel like you are doing something to make a difference in the fight to find a cure. And when you look out over the sea of people who have experienced this terrible disease, whether as a sufferer or a caregiver, you no longer feel so alone.

I have also written letters to my congressmen, requesting that they support ongoing efforts to fund Alzheimer's disease research at the National Institutes of Health. I follow closely the work of our state senators and representatives in fighting for this cause. I was elated to hear that the US Congress approved $425 million for Alzheimer's disease research at the NIH in 2019. I encourage anyone who is affected by this disease to advocate in this way.

Reading these informative books, getting involved with the Alzheimer's Association, and following government developments with regards to Alzheimer's disease helped me in the months and years after Dad's death. The books helped me through my grief. And getting involved in the causes helped me to feel like I was doing something to help others suffering from this disease. It made me feel that Dad's suffering and death were not in vain.

CHAPTER 41

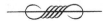

To Take the Test....or Not

After Dad's long journey through Alzheimer's disease, I learned of a test in which you would be able to find out if you were genetically predisposed to getting the disease. The test evaluated whether you have the APOE-e4 Alzheimer's risk gene. It is the first Alzheimer's risk gene and the one with the strongest impact. Having one copy of the APOE-e4 gene increases your risk of having the disease. Having two copies of it, increases it more.

Upon learning about the test, I began doing some soul-searching. Did I want to know if I was going to be like my father and suffer this devastating, debilitating disease? Would my family be better prepared if we knew this ahead of time? Would I be able to put plans in place for my care? I did not know whether I was prepared for this information.

Over the long years of watching Dad decline, I had read many articles stating that Alzheimer's disease was hereditary. The articles stated that those who have a parent, brother, or sister with Alzheimer's are more likely to develop the disease. This was not good news for Sam or me.

I had also read about many steps that one could take to lessen the chances of getting Alzheimer's. A healthy diet, plenty of exercise, brain-stimulating activities like reading, doing crossword puzzles, and learning something new were some of the suggestions to help ward off the disease. I had always eaten healthy and exercised, but I found myself being extra diligent about this when Dad was declining. I began running again, which I had done regularly when I was younger. And I began consciously watching what I was eating to make sure it was very healthy.

I had always been an avid reader during my life. I often referred to myself as a "chain reader," going from one book to another without missing a beat, much like a chain-smoker. So I had that part covered. But I also began doing crossword puzzles and brain-challenging games on my phone every night to keep my brain stimulated.

I read an article in which it claimed that researchers believe that taking ginkgo biloba improves cognitive function because it promotes good blood circulation in the brain and protects the brain from neuronal damage. Out I went to the nearest vitamin store to buy the biggest bottle that I could find, which I split with Sam. We religiously took this supplement every day for years. Until the next study that I read claimed that there was no concrete evidence that ginkgo biloba helped stave off Alzheimer's disease. Next, I read that eating blueberries provided antioxidants that helped with the brain plaque prevalent in Alzheimer's patients. I added blueberries to almost everything I ate.

While I was doing all the preventative measures that were recommended in the many medical articles that I read, there was always the nagging worry that they may not be enough. Dad had always eaten healthy, was a strong proponent of physical exercise, and had done many brain-stimulating activities in his day-to-day living. However, he had developed the disease. Was it something in his gene pool? Was it something that I had inherited?

What would I gain by knowing that I had the Alzheimer's gene? Would it change anything in my life? Would I be able to do anything about it? I decided at the time not to find out. I already worried whenever I misplaced my keys or my wallet. I became concerned each time I forgot something important. And I became upset whenever I could not remember what I had walked into a room for. But was this Alzheimer's disease or just a typical busy life and normal aging?

Over the years since Dad has gone, the genetic testing for the disease has become more prevalent and more accessible with the FDA approving an at-home saliva test for the gene. I still consider taking the test and finding out. But then I think about Dad and how he lived each day to its fullest, always happy and with a positive attitude. Had he known what was ahead for him, he may not have been able to do that. And I am certainly not sure that I would be able to. Sometimes it may be better not knowing what life has in store for you.

CHAPTER 42

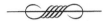

Paying Tribute

After Dads' death, I felt a strong urge to pay tribute to him in some way. I wanted something lasting so that people would know who this great man was and that he was loved. I also wanted to honor the fact that he had fought and served his country. I decided to reach out to the Veterans Administration.

When I told them what I wanted to do, they informed me that since Dad was a veteran, he was entitled to a veteran's marker that would be placed on his grave. Mom and Dad had already purchased a tombstone and had burial plots even before Mom had died. They both had their names and the year of their births engraved on the stone at the time of their purchase. All that would need to be done was to add the year of their deaths. I thought that this was very morbid, but apparently, they wanted to be ready when that day came.

Even though Dad's name was on the tombstone and the year of his death was added, we felt that we would still like to have the veteran's marker. So I gave them all Dad's information, and a few weeks later, they placed his marker next to the tombstone at the head of his grave. It said,

SAMUEL VALENTI
PFC US ARMY
WORLD WAR II
FEB 8, 1920–JAN 23, 2014
BRONZE STAR MEDAL
PURPLE HEART

It was a beautiful memorial marker that Dad would have loved. I was especially happy that they had listed the medals that he was awarded. I felt that it was a wonderful tribute to him.

However, a few months later, Katelyn came up with an even better way to pay tribute to Dad. For years, whenever we would take Dad for the walks that he loved so much, we would go to the Norristown Farm Park. They had a number of scenic trails that we would explore. Along these trails were memorial benches that people had purchased for their deceased loved ones. Dad loved to read the names on the benches. Sometimes he would stop to figure out how old the person who died had been based on the dates on the benches. Many times, he would comment on how much he liked them. So Katelyn suggested we get him one of his own.

We discussed the idea with Sam, and we all agreed it was a terrific idea. I called the parks department and asked how we would go about doing this. They gave me the information that I needed, and we moved forward with our plans.

We all sat down to decide what we wanted inscribed on the bench. Almost all the benches in the park had the deceased person's name along with their birth and death year. But we wanted something different. We agreed that we did not want to have the dates on Dad's bench. We decided on, "In Loving Memory of Sam Valenti." However, we wanted to add a little something extra.

I contacted the parks department and asked if we could have a small plaque attached to the bench with something engraved on it. They told me that there would be an extra charge but that we could do it. We had the perfect idea in mind.

We sent in the form with the engraving that we wanted and the payment for the bench. The parks department told me that it would be ready to be placed in the park in two weeks. Now we just had to find the appropriate spot.

Katelyn struck again. She and Dad used to go to the park together to have their Frosties and fries, and they would sit under a beautiful gazebo. She suggested a spot near the gazebo that was at the top of a hill, overlooking the park. It was the ideal spot.

A few weeks later, the parks department called and told me that the bench and plaque were completed and had been placed in the spot that we requested. We all decided to meet at the park to view it together. As we approached the bench, we commented on how perfect it looked, overlooking the park that Dad had loved so much.

When we arrived, we all read the beautiful tribute, "In Loving Memory of Sam Valenti." And then we all read the plaque. It said, "We Love You! Love, Sam, Maryanne, Jim, Jimmy, and Katelyn. It's So Nice To Get A Whiff Of This Fresh Air." We all laughed as we remembered how many times Dad had repeated that same phrase in the course of our many walks together.

We sat on the bench and reminisced about Dad and what a wonderful person he had been. We talked about the many walks that we had all gone on with him at this park and some of the topics we talked about on those hikes. And how many times he had repeated the same stories over and over as his Alzheimer's disease progressed. But most of all, we talked about how he always had a smile on his face and love in his heart for all of us.

As we left the park that day with tears in our eyes, it was our hope that there would be many people sitting on this bench, over-looking this beautiful park, getting a whiff of the fresh air and know-ing how much Sam Valenti had been loved.

CHAPTER 43

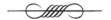

Reflections

Looking back now over the eight years of saying goodbye to my father, I have reflected on many things. And these reflections have caused me to go through a wide range of emotions. As I said at the start of my story, a roller-coaster ride of emotions.

When Dad first started exhibiting the signs of Alzheimer's disease, I was so confused. Was his forgetfulness just normal signs of aging? Was him asking me the same questions repeatedly due to him not paying attention? Was him misplacing things just due to carelessness? I was at a loss as to what was happening.

Once Dad was diagnosed, there was a deluge of emotions. Relief to finally have an answer to the cause of Dad's strange behaviors. Anger that this disease was affecting our family. And sadness that it was not just normal aging, lack of attention, and carelessness. However, the one emotion that prevailed from the day that Dad was diagnosed until he took his last breath was fear—fear of this disease that I knew so little about and what it was going to reduce my father to.

As in many times in my life where there was fear of the unknown, I turned to research. I felt that the more I knew about this debilitating disease, the better equipped I would be to handle it. I would recommend to anyone going through this to read and research as much as you can so that you will be prepared for the many changes that you will observe in your loved one. I would also recommend going onto the Alzheimer's Association website and signing up to receive their newsletter. This is a wonderful resource that offers support and gives updates on the research that is being done. The website also has a 24-7 help line that is available.

One of the emotions that I experienced during Dad's illness that I am embarrassed to admit to was impatience. There were many times that he would ask me the same question repeatedly, and for the first five times, I would answer lovingly. By number six, I would start getting a little testy. By seven or eight, I was ready to scream. Then I am ashamed to admit, I would say, "Dad, I already answered that question" in a rather irritated tone. Dad would look crestfallen, and I would feel awful. I would leave him that day feeling so remorseful and promise myself that the next time I was going to be more patient. And the next time, the whole routine would start over again.

I also learned over the many years of caring for Dad to forgive myself. Caring for someone with Alzheimer's disease requires a great deal of patience. For the most part, I did a decent job. But as I said, I would lose my patience many times and become frustrated. But I started to realize that I am only human and that frustration is a normal and valid response to caring for someone with Alzheimer's disease. I realized that it is okay to feel this way as long as I did not take that frustration out on Dad. When I felt myself getting to a point where I could not take another question or listen to another repetitive story, I would tell myself that I needed a break from him for a while. I would call Sam or Barbara or Carla and ask them to pick up the slack so that I could have a little respite. Then I would come back feeling refreshed and ready, once again, to take on the challenges that this disease presented.

Along with the feelings of impatience came the guilt—guilt that I was not being understanding and tolerant, guilt that I was not doing enough, guilt that I did not want to be a caregiver anymore, and guilt that I felt that way. But I came to realize that while it is normal to feel this emotion, I had to give myself a break. I was there for Dad every step of the way through his Alzheimer's journey. It is important as a caregiver to realize that you have to give yourself credit for everything that you do for your loved one. It is easy to feel guilty for what you are not able to do, but you need to stop and praise yourself once in a while for all that you are doing. It is a very difficult job caring for a loved one who is a shadow of the person that they used to be.

There were many negative emotions experienced throughout this long journey through Dad's illness. However, after Dad's death, I also reflected on the positive experiences that we had along the way. Of course, at the time, I did not appreciate them because I was so bogged down with the responsibilities of caregiving. But looking back, Dad taught us many valuable lessons while he was on this voyage.

One lesson that comes to mind often is appreciation. Dad was always so appreciative of everything that anyone did for him. There was never a time that he did not say, "Thank you, sweetheart" to me or whoever else did something to help him. Even though he was suffering confusion and the loss of his independence each and every day, he always remembered to tell the people around him how much he appreciated what they did for him.

Another lesson was perseverance. Many times when things have not gone well in my life, I have felt like curling up in a ball and not getting out of bed. However, Dad just kept plugging away at life, no matter what it threw at him. He just kept going and going—like the Energizer Bunny.

Perhaps the most important lesson he taught me was kindness. Dad was the epitome of kindness. Again, even as he suffered the humiliation of losing his dignity and independence, even when he knew that he was not the man that he used to be, he never took it out on the people around him. He always remained the kind and caring person that he had been his whole life. I received many texts and e-mails from friends and acquaintances who had known Dad after he passed away, and they all had the same theme. Everyone remarked about the kindhearted and gracious man that he was. It made me so proud.

Dad had taught me many things throughout my life. As I said in the letter that I read to him at his funeral, he taught me how to dance, how to change a tire, how to ride a bike, and how to drive. However, some of the most important things that Dad taught me were during this eight year goodbye. I admire the way he handled his decline, retaining as much of his dignity as he could, never losing sight of the people who were there to help him along the way, and keeping his sense of humor.

This long journey took us all on a wild ride of ups and downs. There were days that we laughed, days that we cried, days that we wanted to scream, and days that we wanted to jump for joy when Dad was able to remember something that he had previously forgotten. It truly was exhausting, rewarding, depressing, awe-inspiring, confusing, and a whole host of other emotions. A roller-coaster ride of emotions.

I reflect on all of this when I am outside in the sunshine—Dad's favorite kind of day. Or when I am listening to our song, "You Make Me Feel Brand New" (not "Highway to Hell"). I think of all that I learned about my father while he bravely fought the battle of Alzheimer's disease as I am going on a long walk in one of the many parks that he and I used to explore. I smile when I realize that he is at peace now and no longer suffering the confusion and disorientation of Alzheimer's disease. And I am thankful for the time that I had with him. And as I am outside enjoying the beautiful day and reflecting on all of this, I think to myself, "It's so nice to get a whiff of this fresh air!"

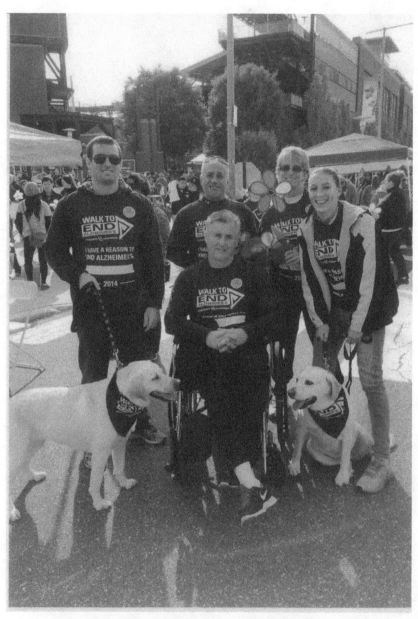

At the Walk to End Alzheimer's in Philadelphia, November 2014. Our group was called "Pappers Pals."

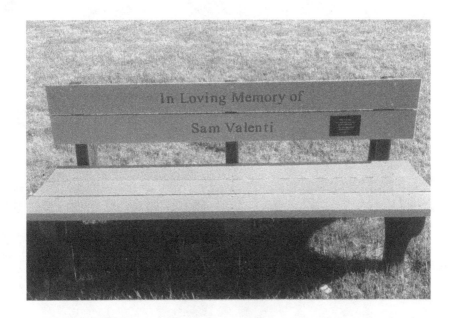

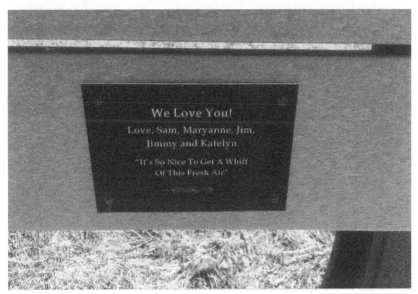

Our tribute to Dad

ACKNOWLEDGMENTS

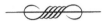

After my father died, I began writing down some of the things that had happened in the last few months of his life. I wanted to always remember the awe-inspiring phenomenon of Dad seeing Mom and his brother and the peacefulness that overcame him in his final days. However, as time went on, I also began writing down some of the many other things that we experienced along the journey of Alzheimer's disease. Somewhere along the way, it started to turn into a book. But it was not until friends and acquaintances started to experience this terrible disease with members of their own families and began turning to me for advice on how to handle it that this book became a very real possibility. And then my friend Ray, who was experiencing Alzheimer's disease with his father, said, "You are a wealth of knowledge on this subject. You should write a book." While I in no way consider myself an expert on this subject, I do feel that I experienced enough of the effects of the disease to offer the support, advice, and comradery that I hope this book will provide to its readers.

I received so much encouragement along the way as I wrote this book. My friends cheered me on and supported me every step of the way. But even more important than the cheering and encouragement during the writing of the book is the unending support they gave me while I was going through this eight-year battle. I will be forever grateful to my dear friends, Laurie Garafola, Mary Feit, Karen Verna, Cathy Dewald, Mel Hauser, Debbie Kresch, Danielle Franco, Judy McKeon, Doug Loughery, and Margaret Loughery. If it were not for their love and support during my many years of sadness and despair in dealing with Dad's decline, I am not sure I would have made it.

They spent countless hours listening to me cry, rant, and repeat the same sad story over and over and never made me feel that I was a burden. Thank you so much, my dear friends.

To my angels sent from God, Barbara and Carla, I cannot possibly thank you enough for being part of Dad's caregiving team. From the day we met both of you, we knew that you would care for Dad and love him. You provided Sam and I with the peace of mind we needed when we could not be there with him all the time. When he was first diagnosed, Sam and I said that we wished we had more siblings to help with the caregiving that was going to be involved in walking this path with Dad. Little did we know that we would be gaining two "sisters" along this journey. We are so thankful for both of you, and you will forever be part of our family. Always know how much Dad loved you.

To my children, words cannot express the admiration and respect that I have for you both in how you handled your grandfather's decline. You were by his side, loving him, and making him feel valued each step of the way. I know that there were times that it was difficult for you to see him in his diminished condition, but you never faltered in your love and care for him. He loved you with all his heart, and you did a wonderful job showing him how much you loved and treasured him. You were the lights of his life.

To my brother and my partner through all this, Mom always used to tell us when we were growing up, "You guys will always have each other. People will come and go in your life, but you need to always be there for each other." We certainly lived up to that, and we were truly a team in this long battle. We worked so well together, ensuring that Dad's needs were always met. You were an amazing son and an exceptional caregiver to our father. I could not have asked for a better ally to fight this battle with. Or for a more remarkable brother. I am so thankful for you.

And finally, to my husband…I was not the easiest person to live with during this eight year journey. You lived every day with my depression, my hopelessness, and my anger at this awful disease. And you continued to love me and be a constant source of support. I will be forever grateful to you for being there for better or for worse…

In this case, there was more "worse" than "better." You were a terrific son-in-law to my father and an incredible husband to me when I needed you the most. I thank God every day for you.

To anyone reading this book who may be able to relate to the effects of this horrendous disease, I hope that some of what I wrote about was a help to you. And I wish for you peace and acceptance. Remember to take care of yourself so that you will be able to take care of your loved one. And let's all pray for a cure for Alzheimer's disease so that others will not have to go through the devastation that this disease brings.

ABOUT THE AUTHOR

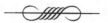

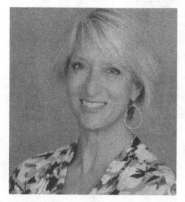

M aryanne V. Scott was born in Pennsylvania to Italian American parents who stressed the importance of family and caring for one another. She grew up in a middle-class household with her younger brother, Sam. Life revolved around family get-togethers and enjoying the simple things that life has to offer. Maryanne graduated from Temple University with a degree in business administration / marketing. She worked for many years for Unisys Corporation until her husband's career brought them to Albany, New York, for six years. At that time, she decided to stay at home to raise her children and work part time as a Teacher's Aide in their school district. Shortly upon returning to Pennsylvania, Maryanne's father developed Alzheimer's disease, and she became his caregiver for eight years while also working part time, raising her two children, and caring for her husband who had a spinal cord injury. Upon her father's death from the disease, she decided to become involved in the crusade to fight this devastating illness. Today she lives in Bucks County, Pennsylvania, with her husband and works as an Educational Assistant in the local school district. She continues to advocate for Alzheimer's disease research by participating in annual Walks to End Alzheimer's and writing to her congressmen, encouraging them to support efforts to fund Alzheimer's research at the National Institutes of Health. It is her dream to see a world without Alzheimer's disease.

CPSIA information can be obtained
at www.ICGtesting.com
Printed in the USA
LVHW051126110521
687090LV00002B/195